Angiography and
Interventional Radiology

Angiography and
Interventional Radiology

Robert J. Rosen, MD

Associate Professor of Radiology
Director, Vascular and Interventional Radiology
New York University Medical Center
New York, New York

John Nosher, MD

Professor of Clinical Radiology
University of Medicine and Dentistry of New Jersey
Robert Wood Johnson Medical School
New Brunswick, New Jersey

J. B. Lippincott Company • Philadelphia
Gower Medical Publishing • New York • London

Distributed in USA and Canada by:
J.B. Lippincott Company
East Washington Square
Philadelphia, PA 19105
USA

Distributed in the rest of the world (except Japan) by:
Gower Medical Publishing
Middlesex House
34-42 Cleveland Street
London W1P 5FB
UK

Distributed in Japan by:
Nankodo Company Ltd.
42-6, Hongo 3-Chome
Bunkyo-Ku
Tokyo 113
Japan

10 9 8 7 6 5 4 3 2 1

Library of Congress Cataloging-in-Publication Data
Nosher, John.
    Angiography and interventional radiography / John
Nosher, Robert J Rosen
        p.   cm.
    Includes bibliographical references and index.
    ISBN 1–56375–003–1
    1. Angiography.   2. Radiology, Interventional.
I. Rosen, Robert J. (Robert Jay), 1951-   . II. Title
    [DNLM: 1. 1. Angiography.   2. Radiography,
Interventional. WG 500 N897a]
RC691.6.A53N67   1991
616.1'0757—dc20
DNLM/DLC
for Library of Congress   91-10562
                                    CIP

British Library Cataloguing in Publication Data
Nosher, John.
    Angiography and interventional radiology.
    1. Humans. Circulatory system. Radiology
    I. Title II. Rosen, Robert J.
    616.130757
    ISBN 1–56375–003–1

Editors: Bill Gabello, Patrick D. O'Neill
Art Director: Jill Feltham
Illustrator: Alan Landau, Seward Hung
Designer: Nava Anav
Layout: Nancy Berliner

Printed in Hong Kong
Produced by Mandarin Offset

7-15-92

CONTENTS

SECTION I:

Diagnostic Angiography

C H A P T E R   O N E

General Angiographic Techniques

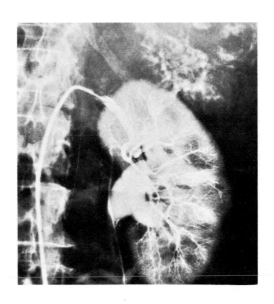

CATHETER PLACEMENT

Over the past 30 years various techniques have been employed to examine blood vessels radiographically. The most widely accepted method involves the placement of small catheters directly into the arterial system under fluoroscopic guidance. Catheter placement is performed using a technique described in 1953 by Seldinger (Fig. 1.1): The artery is punctured percutaneously; a flexible wire, known as a guidewire, is passed through the needle into the vessel; the needle is removed, and a catheter is threaded into the vessel over the wire. Since the guidewire maintains access to the vessel, various catheters can be inserted or exchanged for one another through the same entry site.

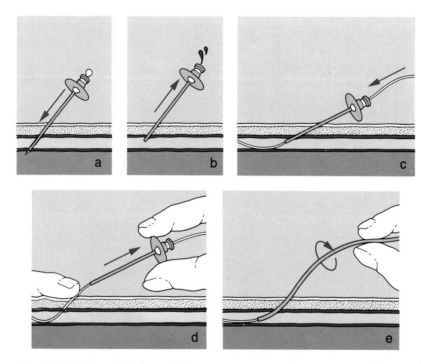

Fig. 1.1 Seldinger technique. *This sequence shows the steps involved in the Seldinger technique for percutaneous catheterization of blood vessels. **a** After the pulse is located by palpation, the skin is prepped and infiltrated with local anesthetic. The vessel is then punctured at a 45° angle through-and-through with a removable stylet needle. **b** The stylet is removed, leaving the hollow outer cannula. The cannula is then gradually withdrawn until a strong spurt of arterial blood indicates intraluminal position. **c** The cannula is tilted to a shallower angle and a soft guidewire is passed through it into the vessel lumen. No resistance should be felt to the passage of the wire. **d** While the guidewire is held in place and manual compression is applied to the entry site, the cannula is withdrawn. **e** The angiographic catheter is then threaded over the guidewire into the vessel, generally with a rotary motion to ease entry. A short dilating catheter is often used prior to insertion of the angiographic catheter. Once the catheter is in the vessel, the guidewire is removed and the catheter is flushed with heparinized saline.*

ENTRY SITES

Certain anatomic locations are favored for access to the vascular system due to their percutaneous accessibility (a palpable pulse is required), their size, and their capability of being compressed directly to seal the opening after catheter removal.

The most common entry sites are the femoral, brachial, and axillary arteries (Fig. 1.2). The femoral artery approach is the most frequently employed, as it is quite safe and provides fairly direct access to most parts of the vascular system.

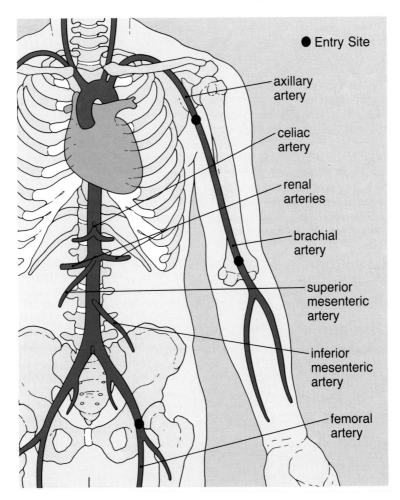

● Entry Site

- axillary artery
- celiac artery
- renal arteries
- brachial artery
- superior mesenteric artery
- inferior mesenteric artery
- femoral artery

Fig. 1.2 Entry sites. *The common entry sites used for angiographic examination (marked by dots).*

CATHETER SELECTION

Once the vascular system has been entered, the selection of a catheter and its positioning depend on the structures to be examined. There are many variations, but the two main categories of angiographic catheters are *flush* and *selective* (Fig. 1.3). Flush catheters, which may be straight or have a preformed "pigtail" tip, have numerous side-holes near the tip designed to deliver a large bolus into a major vessel, such as the aorta or pulmonary artery. Flush-catheter studies show more general anatomic territory, and provide less information about specific organs. Selective catheters, on the other hand, usually have only one opening, or end-hole, at the tip and are designed to be placed into smaller vessels for studies of specific organs (Fig. 1.4). Of the many available shapes and sizes of selective catheters, some, such as the "cobra" curve, are useful for many selective studies, while others are designed to permit catheterization of a specific vessel, such as the gastroduodenal artery. These catheters are radiopaque, and are manipulated under fluoroscopic guidance. With experience, remarkably small distal vessels can be selectively catheterized.

CONTRAST INJECTION

When the catheter has been positioned, contrast is injected at a specific rate and volume, usually with an automatic injector. For flush studies, contrast material is injected at a rapid rate whereas much lower rates of injection are required in selectively catheterized smaller vessels. Rapid sequential films are then taken. General guidelines for injection rates and filming sequences are available in angiographic texts, but these are often modified according to the specific situation at hand. Obtaining high-quality studies safely and routinely requires considerable experience.

COMPLICATIONS

By definition, angiography is an invasive procedure with certain inherent risks: those related to the contrast material, and those arising from the mechanics of insertion and manipulation of catheters within the blood vessels.

Contrast-related risks include allergy (ranging in severity from mild hives to anaphylaxis), renal toxicity, and neurotoxicity. Allergic reactions are not dose-related, whereas toxic effects to the kidneys and nervous system often are. Risks related to catheter insertion and manipulation include vessel occlusion, dissection (intimal injury), perforation, embolization, and hematoma formation at the entry site. Careful technique and experience can reduce but not completely eliminate the occurrence of these complications.

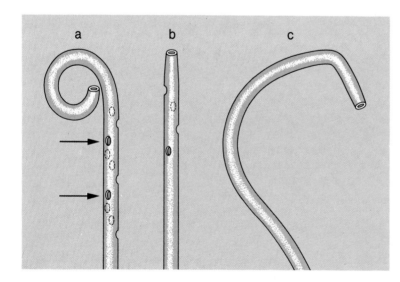

Fig. 1.3 Commonly used angiographic catheters. *a The pigtail catheter is used for high-volume flush studies in large vessels such as the aorta and the pulmonary artery. The pigtail curve is an atraumatic shape that forces most of the contrast to exit the multiple side-holes (arrows) for a uniform bolus. b Another common type of flush catheter is straight with an end-hole and multiple side-holes. The straight configuration and end-hole add some risk of vessel trauma from the jet effect at the tip. c A commonly used catheter for selective study of branch blood vessels, such as the celiac axis, superior mesenteric artery, and renal arteries, is referred to as a cobra curve; the only opening is at the catheter tip.*

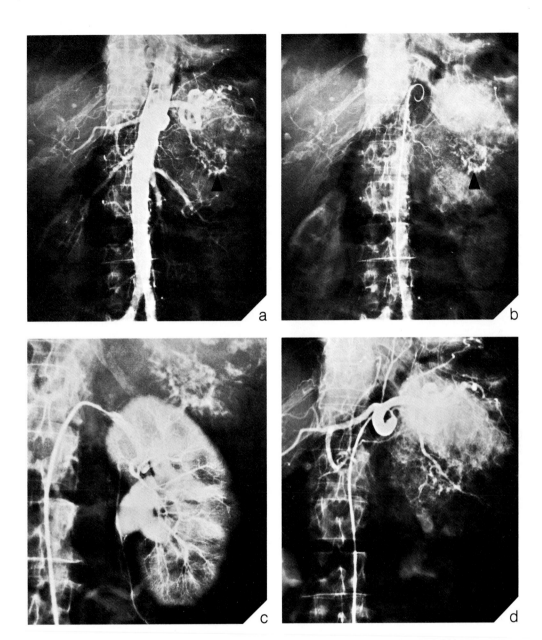

Fig. 1.4 Angiographic evaluation of a mass.
Sequence of studies in the angiographic evaluation of a mass in the left upper quadrant.
a Flush aortogram, performed with a pigtail catheter, shows filling of the aorta and its major abdominal trunks—celiac, SMA, renals, IMA. Some vessels are seen in the region of the calcified mass in the left upper abdomen (arrow). b A late-phase film from the same injection shows the calcification more clearly (arrow).

c In a selective study of the left kidney, performed by inserting a cobra catheter into the left renal artery, the kidney appears normal and unrelated to the mass above it. d In a selective celiac axis study, also performed with a cobra catheter, the numerous pancreatic branches of the splenic artery that supply the hypervascular mass suggest that it originates from the pancreas. At surgery the mass was found to be a pancreatic cystadenoma.

C H A P T E R   T W O

*T*horax

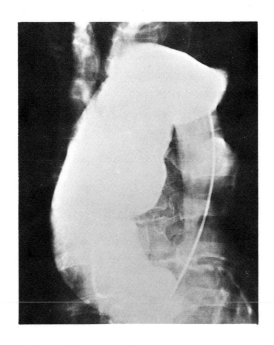

THORACIC AORTOGRAPHY

Thoracic aortography is performed by inserting a flush catheter, usually of the pigtail type, into the root of the aorta by the femoral, the brachial, or the axillary approach (see Fig. 1.2). Rapid injection and filming rates are required for optimal visualization due to the extremely high velocity of flow in this portion of the circulation.

The best single projection for evaluating the thoracic aorta is the right posterior oblique view. This projection throws the arch into profile, whereas on the anteroposterior view, the ascending and descending segments of the arch are superimposed. In addition to the aorta itself, the study usually provides good visualization of the aortic valve and the proximal brachiocephalic vessels.

Thoracic aortography is most frequently indicated for evaluation of suspected aneurysms, aortic dissection, severe atherosclerosis, coarctation, trauma, and masses found on standard chest films and suspected of being vascular in nature.

The examination is generally quite safe. In addition to the risks of any angiogram, there is, however, the danger of neurologic injury, since the injection site is proximal to the origins of the brachiocephalic vessels.

Atherosclerotic Disease

Atherosclerosis commonly involves the thoracic aorta, but hemodynamically significant stenosis is extremely rare. The disease process may become clinically significant by involving the origins of the brachiocephalic vessels, with resultant neurologic sequelae or ischemic symptoms in the upper extremities (Fig. 2.1). Ulcerated plaques may also serve as a nidus for embolization to almost any part of the circulation. Aneurysmal disease of the thoracic aorta (see below) is another common manifestation of atherosclerosis.

Aneurysmal Disease

Aneurysmal disease, which may involve any segment of the thoracic aorta, most commonly occurs in the ascending and descending segments, the transverse segment being relatively spared.

Atherosclerotic aneurysms are by far the most frequent type, but other disorders may cause aneurysmal dilation or even rupture of the thoracic aorta. These less-common causes should be suspected when there is selective involvement of the aortic root and ascending segment. Syphilis and connective tissue disorders such as Marfan's syndrome both result in degeneration of the media (cystic medial necrosis), which is the pathologic process underlying the dilation. When the aortic root becomes severely dilated, the valve may be affected, resulting in aortic insufficiency (Fig. 2.2).

Atherosclerotic aneurysms are extremely variable in their appearance, ranging from long and fusiform to discrete and saccular. Calcification is often seen in the wall, and the margins of the lumen may show diffuse irregularity representing ulcerated plaques or a smooth featureless contour when laminated thrombus is present. Most of these aneurysms are asymptomatic and are discovered as a mass on routine chest films (Fig. 2.3). When a patient presents with chest or back pain, leakage or impending rupture must be suspected and urgent evaluation and therapy carried out. Rupture of the aneurysm, associated with a high mortality rate, may occur into the pleural space, the mediastinum, or the pericardium (Fig. 2.4).

Aortic Dissection

Aortic dissection, sometimes referred to as dissecting aneurysm, is a process involving disruption of the aortic intimal lining and dissection of blood between the layers of the vessel wall. Although the exact mechanism of dissection is not entirely understood, a primary degeneration of the vessel wall, commonly associated with significant systemic hypertension, is thought to be involved. Part of the nonsurgical management consists of decreasing the blood pressure.

Dissections may be localized or extend below the diaphragm as far distally as the femoral arteries. The major complications of this process are acute aortic valvular insufficiency, free rupture of the vessel wall, and shearing of branch vessels resulting in ischemia of almost any part of the body. The most common presenting symptom is pain: often sudden, severe tearing chest pain radiating to the back. In other cases ischemic complications, such as stroke, renal or intestinal infarction, or acute ischemia of the extremities may be seen. Therapy, usually involving surgery to repair the intimal tear, must be initiated rapidly, along with measures to reduce the blood pressure.

The angiographic hallmarks of dissection are opacification of more than one parallel lumen and visualization of the intimal flap, which appears as a sharply outlined linear lucency within the contrast-filled lumen (Fig. 2.5). In some cases catheterization by the femoral route is ruled out due to discontinuity of the lumen at this level with the "true" lumen of the thoracic aorta. A right axillary approach may be required in these cases to catheterize the aortic root. Thoracic dissections are commonly classified according to the anatomic segment involved: type 1 involves the entire thoracic aorta starting at the root; type 2 involves only the ascending segment; and type 3 begins just beyond the origin of the left subclavian artery and extends distally. The abdominal aorta is usually studied at the same time to determine the distal extent of the dissection process. Often a second intimal disruption, known as a reentry flap, occurs distally where the false lumen has ruptured and again communicates with the true lumen.

Trauma

Penetrating injuries that carry an extremely high mortality rate can involve any portion of the thoracic aorta. Angiographic visualization of extravasation is almost unheard of, since this is generally associated with rapid cardiovascular collapse.

Blunt trauma tends to produce a specific type of injury to the thoracic aorta. The transverse segment of the aorta, just beyond the origin of the left subclavian artery in the region of the ligamentum arteriosum, is a common site of injury, usually involving a disruption of varying degrees of severity of the aortic wall. This type of injury is generally associated with chest trauma in motor vehicle accidents; fractures of the sternum and upper ribs are often seen in association with this type of injury. Complete transection of the aorta may occur, leading in most cases to almost immediate death; in some, however, the integrity of the adventitia, a very strong layer of the vessel wall, may prevent free hemorrhage and allow survival (Fig. 2.6). An important clue to the presence of this injury, known as traumatic pseudoaneurysm or aortic transection, is widening of the upper mediastinal contour on the initial chest film. In a patient with a history of severe chest trauma, this finding indicates the need for emergency aortography, as the risk of delayed free rupture is extremely high in the period immediately following injury. In some patients the diagnosis of pseudoaneurysm, missed at the time of injury, may be picked up as a mass on a routine chest film many years later (Fig. 2.7).

Thoracic Outlet Syndrome

The arteries, veins, and nerves of the upper extremity are subject to extrinsic compression at several specific anatomic sites. Typically, compression is associated with symptoms of pain, abnormal sensation, weakness, and occasionally atrophy or even frank ischemia of the extremity. This symptom complex is known as thoracic outlet syndrome. Clinical tests and maneuvers can elicit characteristic findings, such as positional loss of distal pulses, but arteriography or venography are often needed to confirm the diagnosis prior to surgery.

Arterial compression may be evaluated on an aortic arch study or on a selective subclavian arteriogram. The initial study is performed with the arm in neutral position; repeat studies use various positions designed to demonstrate extrinsic compression by muscles, tendons, or bony structures (Fig. 2.8).

Venous compression may also occur, with symptoms of arm swelling and venous engorgement; thrombosis may develop also as a result of the extrinsic compression. The veins are studied by simply injecting contrast through a vein in the hand or arm (see Chapter 5 on venography of the extremities).

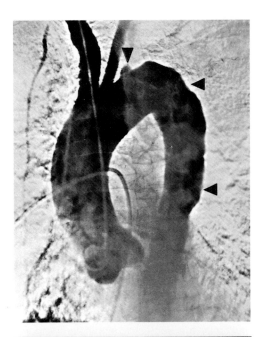

Fig. 2.1 Atherosclerosis of aortic arch.
Subtraction film in the right posterior oblique projection of the thoracic aorta in a 62-year-old man with symptoms of exertional pain in the left arm. Note the occlusion of the proximal left subclavian artery (arrow 1), as well as diffuse atherosclerotic disease of the transverse and descending thoracic aorta (arrows 2).

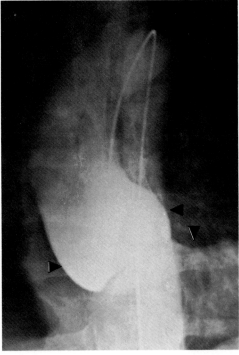

Fig. 2.2 Aortic aneurysm (Marfan's syndrome). *A 53-year-old man with known Marfan's syndrome presented with decreasing exercise tolerance and a loud murmur of aortic insufficiency. Thoracic aortogram (anteroposterior view) demonstrates aneurysmal dilation of the aortic root and the ascending segment (arrows 1) typical of the aneurysmal disease seen in connective tissue disorders. The contrast-filled left ventricle (arrow 2) reflects severe incompetence of the aortic valve.*

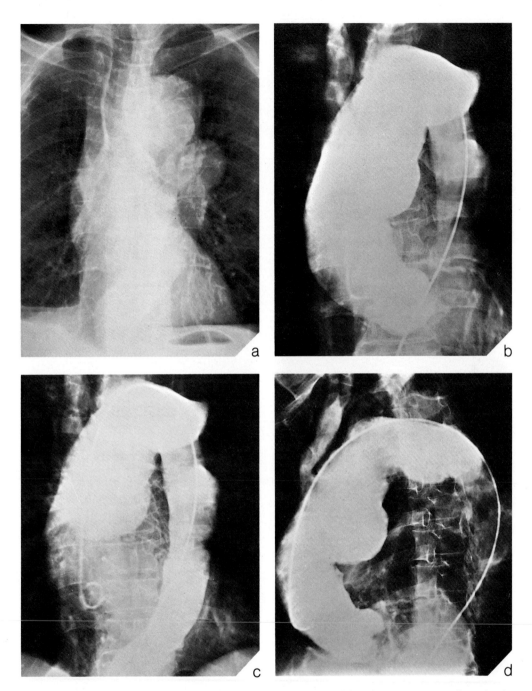

Fig. 2.3 Asymptomatic aortic aneurysm.
a An 80-year-old man was found to have a mediastinal mass on routine chest x-ray that appeared related to the aortic shadow.
b, c Thoracic aortograms in the AP projection show a long segment of severe aneurysmal disease involving the transverse and proximal descending aorta. d A repeat injection in the right posterior oblique projection demonstrates the anatomy more clearly, particularly the relationship of the aneurysm to the brachiocephalic vessels.

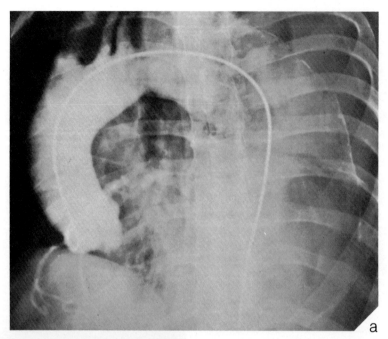

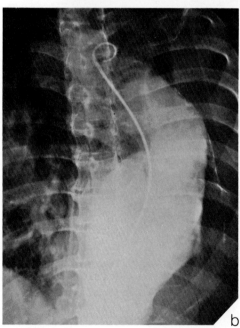

Fig. 2.4 Ruptured aortic aneurysm. *A 72-year-old man presented in shock following an episode of severe "tearing" chest pain. On the plain chest film (not shown), the left hemithorax was completely opacified.* **a, b** *An emergency thoracic aortogram in the right posterior oblique projection demonstrates a huge descending thoracic aneurysm which was rupturing into the left chest. Curvilinear calcification is seen outlining the wall of this massive aneurysm. The patient died during attempted surgical repair.*

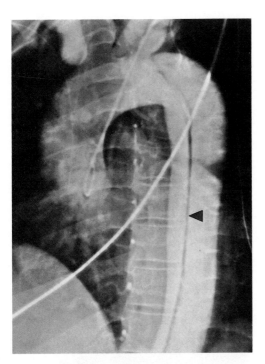

Fig. 2.5 Aortic dissection. *A 33-year-old man with a long-standing history of severe hypertension was admitted with severe chest pain radiating to the back. Thoracic aortogram obtained via the axillary approach demonstrates the typical findings of a type 3 aortic dissection. The sharply outlined lucency (arrow) represents the intimal flap separating the true and false lumina.*

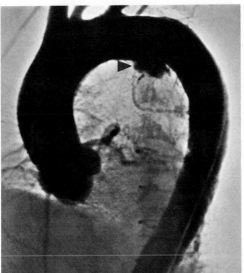

Fig. 2.6 Traumatic aortic paeudoaneurysm. *A 58-year-old man was admitted with multiple injuries, including severe sternal trauma, sustained in a motor vehicle accident. Widening of the upper mediastinal contour noted on his admission chest film (not shown) indicated the need for emergency aortography. The aortogram in the right posterior oblique projection demonstrates a saccular outpouching just beyond the origin of the left subclavian artery (arrow)—a finding typical of traumatic pseudoaneurysm. The intact adventitial layer prevented free rupture.*

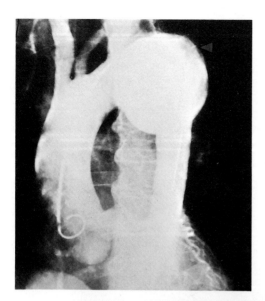

Fig. 2.7 Chronic traumatic pseudo-aneurysm. *In some patients the diagnosis of aortic transection is missed at the time of initial injury. The resulting chronic pseudoaneurysm (arrow) may be picked up as a mass on routine chest examination many years later. In this patient, trauma occurred 20 years previously. Surgery is generally recommended, as delayed rupture is a constant threat.*

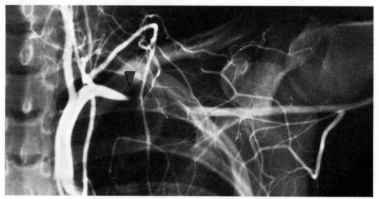

Fig. 2.8 Thoracic outlet syndrome. *A 15-year-old girl presented with complaints of abnormal sensation and weakness in the left hand, suggestive of thoracic outlet syndrome. A selective subclavian arteriogram (not shown), obtained with the arm in neutral position, showed no abnormalities. On abduction of the arm, extrinsic compression to the point of occlusion (arrow) of the subclavian artery becomes evident.*

PULMONARY ANGIOGRAPHY

Pulmonary angiography is performed by passing a catheter through the venous circulation and the right heart and into the pulmonary arteries where the contrast injection is made. Its most important application by far is in the diagnosis of pulmonary embolism. Other available studies, including radionuclide lung scanning, can suggest the diagnosis, but direct pulmonary angiography is universally considered the definitive study to confirm the diagnosis (Figs. 2.9–2.11). Since many clinical conditions can mimic pulmonary embolism (Fig. 2.12), and anticoagulation therapy carries significant risk, diagnostic specificity is extremely important.

Although contrast injection into the right atrium or the main pulmonary artery has been employed in performing this study, most angiographers now prefer more selective injections into the right or left pulmonary arteries. The radionuclide lung scan results serve as a guide to the areas of highest suspicion. Selective injections provide the highest-quality images, which are essential in finding small emboli in branch vessels. Oblique and magnification views may also be necessary to clarify questionable findings. The sine qua non of pulmonary embolus on an angiogram is visualization of a lucent filling defect within a contrast-filled vessel. Poor filling, "cut-off" vessels, and areas of apparently decreased perfusion are all nonspecific findings.

While pulmonary angiography involves certain risks, overemphasis of these risks can result in underutilization of an important diagnostic modality. Cardiac arrhythmias—particularly premature ventricular contractions—commonly occur as the catheter is passed through the right side of the heart, but are nearly always transient and generally require no specific therapy. Certain patients with irritable myocardium or preexisting heart blocks may be at increased risk. Acute right heart failure (cor pulmonale) is another risk, nearly always associated with severe preexisting pulmonary hypertension. For this reason, pulmonary arterial pressures are usually measured directly at the time of catheterization. If significant elevation is discovered, the injection rate and volume may be reduced or the study deferred.

Other indications for performing pulmonary arteriography include its occasional use in preoperative evaluation of tumor encasement in patients with neoplasms (an indication of non-resectability) as well as its use in demonstrating pulmonary arteriovenous malformations (AVMs). These are uncommon except in patients with Rendu–Osler–Weber syndrome (Fig. 2.13). In the latter case, pulmonary AVMs may be clinically significant for two reasons: (1) if large or multiple, they may markedly reduce systemic oxygenation; and (2) they may result in paradoxical systemic embolism due to loss of the normal filter of the pulmonary capillary bed. Brain abscess is the most dangerous complication of this event. Transcatheter embolization using flow-guided detachable balloons provides an extremely effective nonsurgical alternative to surgical resection of the involved portion of lung.

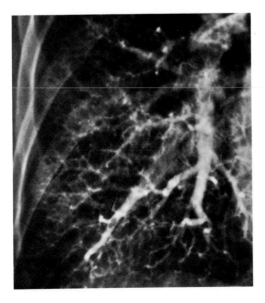

Fig. 2.9 Pulmonary embolus. *Pulmonary angiography represents the "gold standard" in the diagnosis of pulmonary embolism. Findings can be quite subtle when the emboli are small and lodged in peripheral branches, but visualization of a lucent filling defect (arrow) within a contrast-filled pulmonary artery is diagnostic. In some cases, oblique films or magnification views are required to make the diagnosis.*

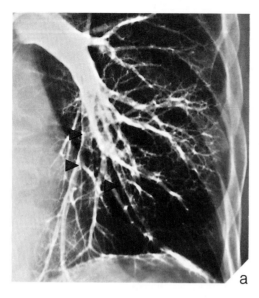

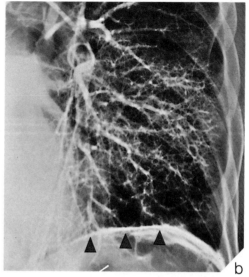

Fig. 2.10 Pulmonary emboli. *A 29-year-old man presented with acute shortness of breath and severe left-sided pleuritic pain. Lung scan (not shown) demonstrated a perfusion defect at the left base, and the chest film (not shown) was within normal limits. **a** A selective left pul-* *monary arteriogram reveals several filling defects in lower lobe branch vessels (arrows). **b** A later-phase film shows marked pleural hyperemia at the lung base (arrows), an unusual finding.*

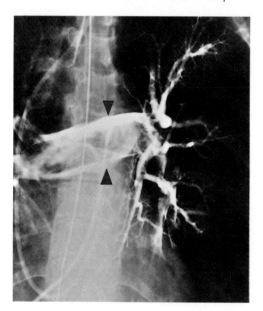

Fig. 2.11 Pulmonary embolus. *Massive pulmonary embolism may result in shock or even sudden death. The only effective therapy for the most severe cases is emergency surgical emborectomy. This case represents a saddle embolus, demonstrated as a huge, lucent filling defect (arrows) in the main pulmonary artery, as well as in both right and left pulmonary arteries.*

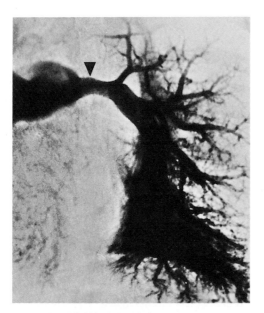

Fig. 2.12 Carcinoma mimicking pulmonary embolism. *A 58-year-old woman presented with symptoms of recurrent pulmonary embolism. A perfusion scan (not shown) revealed decreased flow to the left lung. The arteriogram shows narrowing of the proximal left main pulmonary artery (arrow). Eventually, the encasement was determined to be due to a large central bronchogenic carcinoma.*

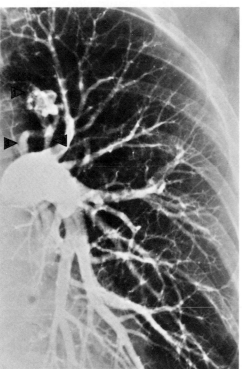

Fig. 2.13 Pulmonary arteriovenous malformation. *A 48-year-old woman with known Rendu–Osler–Weber syndrome presented with increasing dyspnea on exertion and several lobulated parenchymal soft tissue densities on chest radiography (not shown). A left pulmonary arteriogram demonstrates an arteriovenous malformation in the upper lobe (arrow 1) fed by a pulmonary artery branch (arrow 2) and drained by a single pulmonary vein (arrow 3). It was successfully treated by selective embolization using a detachable balloon.*

BRONCHIAL ARTERIOGRAPHY

Selective angiography of the bronchial arteries, small systemic vessels that supply the lung parenchyma and tracheobronchial tree, is technically difficult. It is most often employed in patients with severe hemoptysis in whom all other studies, including bronchoscopy, have failed to clarify the site of bleeding. In addition to actual extravasation, the study may demonstrate areas of abnormal hypervascularity due to chronic inflammation, such as in severe tuberculosis and cystic fibrosis, or even arteriovenous malformation (Fig. 2.14). Embolization may be employed to control hemoptysis nonsurgically.

The main risk of bronchial angiography is neurologic injury related to inadvertent injection of the anterior spinal artery supplying the thoracic spinal cord. This vessel may originate from the bronchial artery trunk or from combined bronchial–intercostal trunks.

SUPERIOR VENA CAVA

Venography of the superior vena cava (SVC) is most frequently indicated in the evaluation of suspected "superior vena cava syndrome." This symptom complex is associated with obstruction of the SVC and includes head, neck, and periorbital edema, venous distension, cyanosis, and, in some cases, syncope. By far the most common cause of obstruction is mediastinal tumor, which either invades or severely compresses the vein. This syndrome may also be seen with mediastinal fibrosis or massive mediastinal adenopathy of benign origin.

The SVC can be studied from an intravenous arm injection, which usually suffices if there is SVC obstruction. Typical findings include peripheral venous engorgement and filling of numerous collateral venous pathways in the neck and chest wall (Fig. 2.15). These collaterals are seen in all but the most acute obstructions. If the SVC is patent or incompletely occluded, a peripheral venous injection produces poor opacification due to a large volume of unopacified blood inflow. Alternative methods of study include passing a catheter from the arm into the subclavian vein or SVC, as well as simultaneous contrast injection into both arms

Aortography may be performed to evaluate abnormalities of the abdominal aorta itself (aneurysm, dissection), or as a general survey of the intraabdominal organs. The study is performed by inserting a flush catheter into the abdominal aorta by one of three approaches: femoral, axillary, or translumbar.

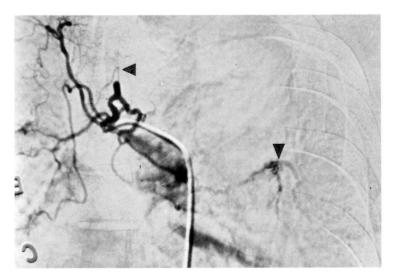

Fig. 2.14 Bronchial arteriovenous fistula. *A 37-year-old man presented with several episodes of massive hemoptysis. A selective injection of the bronchial trunk shows branches to the left and right lungs. Note the presence of a small arteriovenous fistula between the branches of a left bronchial artery and a pulmonary artery (arrow 1). Also note filling of the anterior spinal artery (arrow 2), which may share a common trunk with the bronchial circulation. The hairpin shape and midline position is characteristic of this critically important vessel.*

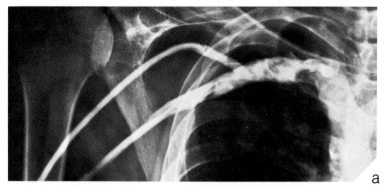

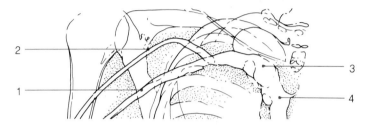

a

2
1

3
4

1 Basilic vein	5 Bronchogenic carcinoma
2 Cephalic vein	6 Subclavian vein
3 Subclavian vein	7 Venous collaterals
4 Superior vena cava	

Fig. 2.15 Normal subclavian venogram/ SVC syndrome.
a Study of right subclavian vein and superior vena cava from right antecubital vein contrast injection. Note normal filling of the basilic and cephalic veins, which then fill the subclavian vein and finally the normal superior vena cava. The lucent defects within the contrast-filled subclavian vein represent inflow of unopacified blood from venous tributaries. b A similar upper extremity venogram performed on a patient with superior vena cava syndrome due to a large bronchogenic carcinoma in the right lung (arrow 5). Note the complete obstruction of the subclavian vein (arrow 6) as well as filling of venous collaterals (arrow 7) bypassing the obstructed superior vena cava.

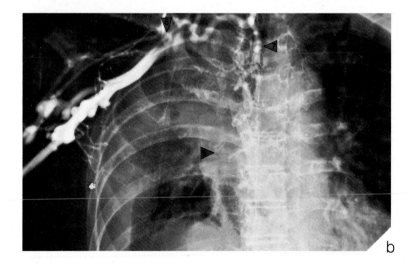

b

*A*bdominal Aortography and Venacavography

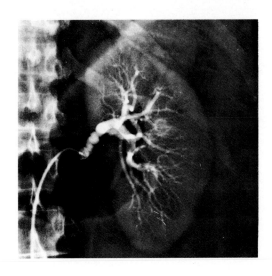

DISORDERS OF THE ABDOMINAL AORTA

Aneurysmal Disease

The diagnosis of abdominal aortic aneurysm is generally made by physical examination, and confirmed by ultrasound or CT (Fig. 3.1). Angiography is used to provide a road map for the surgeon, showing the anatomic extent of the aneurysm, and its relationship to important branch vessels, particularly the renal arteries (Fig. 3.2).

Occlusive Atherosclerotic Disease

Atherosclerosis of the abdominal aorta affects the infrarenal segment most commonly, with associated involvement of the iliac vessels. Findings range from localized plaques, which may ulcerate and embolize distally, to severe narrowing, or even complete occlusion (Figs. 3.3–3.5). When it develops gradually, even complete occlusion of the infrarenal aorta or iliac vessels is remarkably well tolerated by most patients owing to the enormous reserve of potential collateral circulation in the abdomen and pelvis. The Leriche syndrome is the clinical complex associated with aortic occlusion, which consists of buttock and thigh claudication, impotence in males, and absent femoral pulses.

Aortic Dissection

Aortic dissection is described in detail in the previous chapter. This disruption of the intima may be due to intrinsic disease of the vessel wall (atherosclerosis, medial necrosis, arteritis) or trauma (including iatrogenic). Most dissections begin in the thoracic aorta (see Fig. 2.5), but may extend to involve the abdominal aorta and its branches. The angiographic hallmarks of dissection are the "intimal flap" and the presence of more than one lumen (Fig. 3.6).

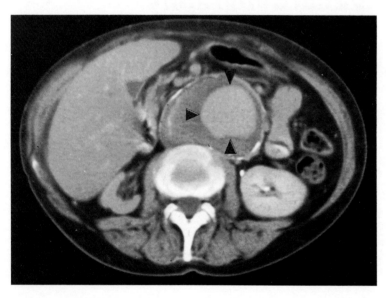

Fig. 3.1 Abdominal aortic aneurysm. *CT examination of a patient with an abdominal aortic aneurysm demonstrates the contrast-filled lumen (arrows) as well as the laminated thrombus. Though this examination clearly demonstrates the relationship of the aorta to surrounding organs, the transverse orientation can be misleading at times, particularly when attempting to determine the relationship of the aneurysm to the renal arteries.*

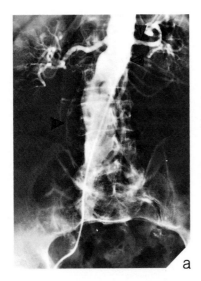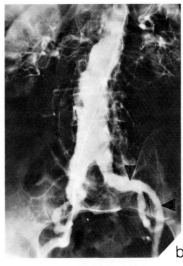

a   b

Fig. 3.2 Abdominal aortic aneurysm. *a Abdominal aortogram of 79-year-old male who presented with a pulsatile abdominal mass. The catheter has been inserted from the femoral artery, and the injection made at the level of the renal arteries (arrow 1). Note the presence of a "neck" (arrow 2) between the renal artery origin and the beginning of the aneurysm. Also note the presence of a thin curvilinear calcification (arrow 3), which shows the true outer wall of the aneurysm. The space between this calcification and the lumen opacified by contrast represents mural thrombus. b As in most abdominal aortic aneurysms, the dilation extends into both common iliac arteries (arrow 1), while the external iliac arteries (arrow 2) are of relatively normal caliber.*

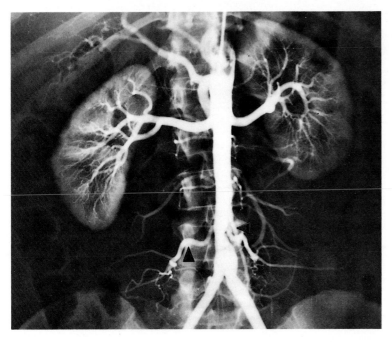

Fig. 3.3 Aortic atherosclerotic plaque. *Aortogram of a 44-year-old woman who presented complaining of claudication in both lower extremities, and was found to have absent femoral pulses bilaterally. The examination was performed therefore via an axillary approach. This midstream aortogram demonstrates a normal upper abdominal aorta and iliac segments; however, there is a large irregular plaque involving the left lateral aspect of the lower abdominal aorta (arrow 1). The hypertrophied lumbar arteries just above this level (arrow 2) confirm the hemodynamic significance of this lesion. This type of lesion often progresses to complete lower aortic occlusion, as is seen in Figure 3.5.*

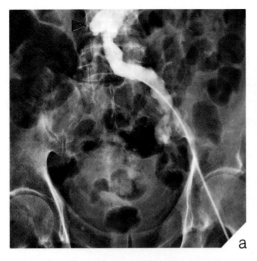

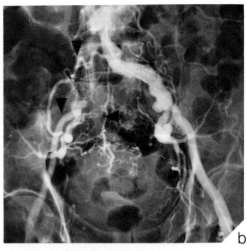

Fig. 3.4 Common iliac artery obstruction. *A 71-year-old patient with a known abdominal aortic aneurysm, and an absent right femoral pulse.* ***a*** *This flush pelvic injection demonstrates aneurysmal disease of the lower abdominal aorta and the left common iliac artery. The right common iliac artery is com-* *pletely occluded* (arrow) *at its origin from the aorta.* ***b*** *A slightly later phase film demonstrates prompt reconstitution of the external iliac artery* (arrow 1) *by the numerous collateral pathways, including the lumbar* (arrow 2) *and middle sacral arteries* (arrow 3).

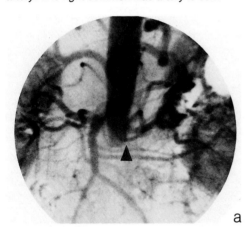

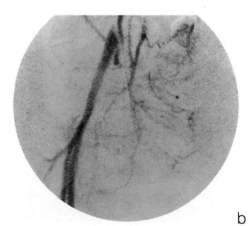

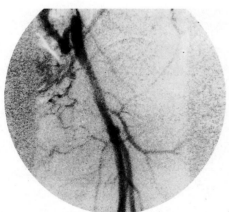

Fig. 3.5 Aortic occlusion with Leriche syndrome. ***a*** *A 57-year-old man with the classic symptoms of Leriche syndrome (buttock and thigh claudication, impotence). Absent femoral pulses were noted on physical examination. A digital intravenous examination demonstrates complete occlusion of the abdominal aorta just below the level of the renal arterial origins* (arrow). ***b, c*** *These images demonstrate the collateral reconstitution of* ***b*** *right and* ***c*** *left external iliac and common femoral arteries. This type of intravenous examination is considerably safer and far easier to perform than transaxillary or translumbar aortography in the evaluation of this type of occlusive disease.*

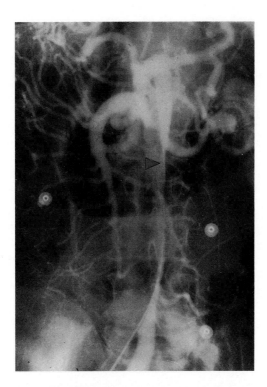

Fig. 3.6 Aortic dissection. *A patient with a long-standing history of hypertension presented with abdominal and back pain of sudden onset. The aortogram demonstrates the bizarre appearance of the aortic lumen, which exhibits sharply tapered narrowing (arrow), and failure of filling of the right renal artery from the main lumen. This type of dissection usually originates in the thoracic aorta, and may result in disastrous clinical sequelae due to ischemia of any of the abdominal viscera.*

RENAL VASCULAR DISEASE

Aortography is frequently employed to investigate acute or chronic obstructions of the renal arterial circulation. Chronic obstruction of the main renal artery is commonly encountered in atherosclerosis. Plaques can severely narrow the vessel lumen at its origin from the abdominal aorta, or there may be stenoses within the renal artery itself (Fig. 3.7). The most common clinical presentation of this type of lesion is uncontrollable hypertension. If the occlusive disease is bilateral and severe enough, frank renal insufficiency may occur. Fibromuscular dysplasia is a distinctive lesion generally found in younger patients that also causes obstruction of renal arterial flow. It appears angiographically as a web-like stenosis, or a series of tight stenoses producing a "beaded" appearance (Fig. 3.8). The lesion is often bilateral and may be encountered in blood vessels in other parts of the body of these same patients.

Acute renal artery occlusion is usually manifested clinically as renal infarction. The clinical symptoms include flank pain, nausea and vomiting, fever, and, in some cases, hematuria. Acute occlusion may be due to aortic dissection, embolic disease, or thrombosis of a previously stenotic artery (Fig. 3.9).

Renal vein thrombosis is encountered in both children and adults. In children it is generally associated with severe dehydration and a poor prognosis. In adults there are numerous causes including generalized systemic disorders as well as renal inflammatory disease.

Acute renal vein occlusion may result in hemorrhagic infarction, while gradual renal vein thrombosis may be well tolerated if there is time for collateral drainage to develop. Renal vein thrombosis may be seen in association with the nephrotic syndrome. The renal venogram is diagnostic, demonstrating thrombus within the vein (Fig. 3.10).

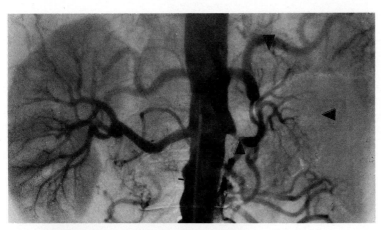

Fig. 3.7 Renal artery stenosis causing hypertension. *A subtraction film from a flush aortogram that demonstrates a tight proximal stenosis of the left renal artery (arrow 1). The left kidney is considerably smaller than the right one due to long-standing impairment of blood flow (arrows 2). This type of lesion can be treated by bypass surgery or balloon angioplasty. If the kidney has been damaged too severely by chronic ischemia ("end stage"), nephrectomy may be the only treatment.*

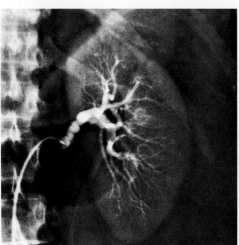

Fig. 3.8 Fibromuscular dysplasia. *A selective left renal arteriogram of a young woman with severe hypertension. The study demonstrates a series of band-like stenoses in the midportion of the main renal artery, a finding characteristic of fibromuscular dysplasia. This type of lesion is encountered most often in young women, and is often bilateral.*

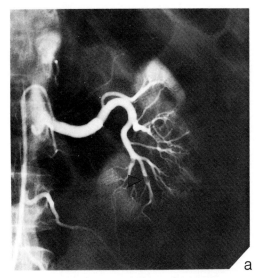

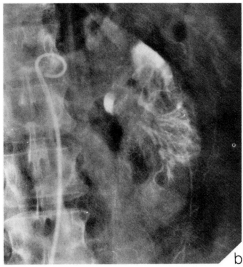

Fig. 3.9 Renal arterial emboli. *a Small filling defects (arrow) typical of emboli within intralobar branches of the renal artery are demonstrated on this selective left renal arteriogram of a 57-year-old woman. The patient presented with long-standing rheumatic mitral valvular dis-* *ease, and the acute onset of left flank pain and microscopic hematuria. b The late-phase film shows a patchy nephrogram, with stasis in the embolized areas. Since the renal arterial bed is an "end circulation," acute arterial occlusions generally lead to infarction.*

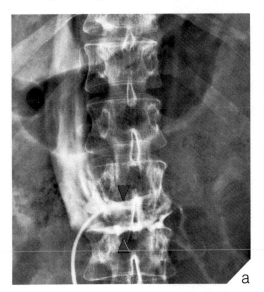

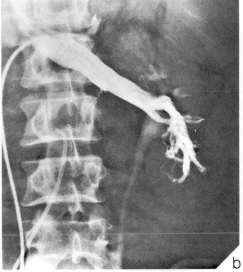

Fig. 3.10 Acute renal vein thrombosis. *a A selective left renal venogram of a 50-year-old man with a long history of multiple myeloma. The patient presented with acute onset of flank pain and hematuria. The venogram demonstrates a large filling defect (arrows) within the* *main renal vein, representing acute renal vein thrombosis. b A normal left renal venogram for purposes of comparison. Note that normally there is poor filling of the peripheral branches due to arterial inflow.*

PELVIC ANGIOGRAPHY

Pelvic hemorrhage due to trauma, surgery, or tumor may be massive; finding the source surgically is notoriously difficult. Pelvic angiography and selective embolization have often proved to be life-saving in such cases (Fig. 3.11).

Arteriovenous malformations occur infrequently, but are found relatively commonly in the pelvis, generally supplied by branches of the hypogastric arteries as well as other pelvic vessels (Fig. 3.12). These lesions tend to progress steadily, and have a marked tendency to recur after attempted surgi-

cal excision or ligation of feeding vessels. A complete angiographic evaluation to determine the extent of a lesion and the involvement of feeding vessels is mandatory prior to any attempted therapy. Recent advances in transcatheter embolization techniques, particularly the use of liquid agents, have allowed this to be used increasingly as a primary therapeutic modality with encouraging preliminary results.

Aside from investigating such specific vascular abnormalities, angiography is not often used in studying the pelvic organs.

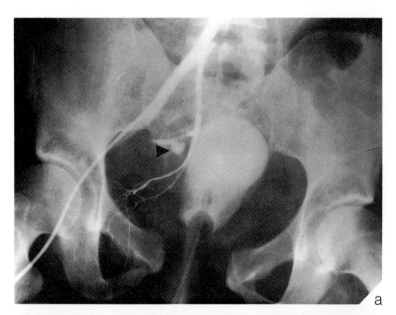

a

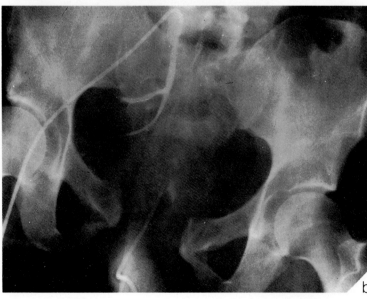

b

Fig. 3.11 Hypogastric artery laceration. *a* This patient sustained massive injuries in an automobile accident, including a severe diastasis injury of the pelvis. Uncontrolled hemorrhage resulted. An emergency arteriogram demonstrates extravasation from a branch of the right hypogastric artery (arrow). *b* Following transcatheter embolization of the traumatized branch, no further extravasation is seen. The patient could then be stabilized clinically.

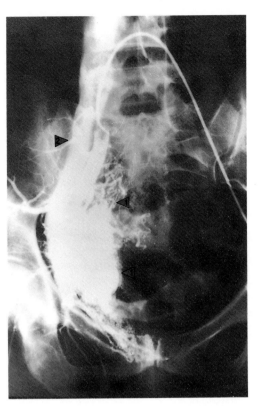

Fig. 3.12 Pelvic arteriovenous malformation.
A hypogastric arteriogram demonstrates a large pelvic arteriovenous malformation (arrows 1). Note the rapid shunting into the iliac vein (arrow 2). This 45-year-old woman presented with lower abdominal pain, and a pulsatile mass on pelvic examination. These lesions are difficult to treat because they are supplied by numerous feeding vessels, and have a marked tendency to progress and recur.

VENACAVOGRAPHY

Leg venography usually allows visualization of the venous system up to the level of the iliac veins. In order to study the inferior vena cava, direct catheterization via a femoral vein puncture is required. Inferior venacavography is performed in the evaluation of thromboembolic disease, to investigate unexplained lower extremity edema, and prior to surgery for large tumors that may be invading, compressing, or otherwise involving the inferior vena cava.

It is normal to see certain filling defects in the contrast-filled inferior vena cava which represent inflow of unopacified blood from various tributary veins, including the iliac, renal, and, sometimes, the hepatic veins. Usually these filling defects appear to change in configuration from one film to the next in the angiographic series (Fig. 3.13). Occasionally, it may be difficult to exclude a true filling defect, such as a blood clot (Fig. 3.14), or extension of tumor thrombus, from the renal vein orifice. In such cases, careful selective catheterization of the tributary vein in question may be required. It is important to keep in mind that the vena cava is a relatively slow-flow system, which may be markedly affected by changes in inspiration or intraabdominal pressure.

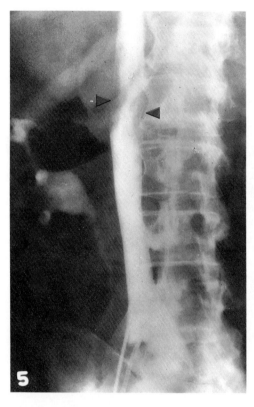

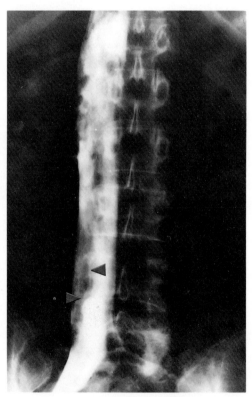

Fig. 3.13 Normal inferior venacavogram. *This normal inferior venacavogram demonstrates the characteristic rather featureless appearance of the vessel. The two poorly defined filling defects (arrows) at the L1 vertebral body level represent the areas of inflow of unopacified blood from each renal vein. The poor definition of these defects as well as the changeability from one film to another allows them to be distinguished from fixed defects, as would be seen with thrombus.*

Fig. 3.14 Thrombus in inferior vena cava. *An inferior venacavogram performed from the right iliac vein demonstrates a large radiolucent filling defect occupying the entire length of the vessel. Note the sharply marginated contours (arrows), which were constant on all films; this would not be characteristic of a flow-related defect and represents a large thrombus.*

*S*elective Abdominal Studies

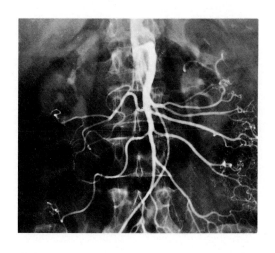

Selective angiography is performed by inserting preshaped catheters into branches of the aorta under fluoroscopic guidance. Much more detailed images of individual abdominal organs are obtained with these selective contrast injections than with a simple flush aortogram.

SELECTIVE VISCERAL ANGIOGRAPHY

The Visceral Circulation

The three major aortic branches that supply the gastrointestinal (GI) tract in the abdomen are the celiac axis, the superior mesenteric artery, and the inferior mesenteric artery. Normal selective celiac axis, SMA, and IMA angiograms are shown in Figs. 4.1–4.3. As in any angiographic study, it is necessary to see the entire sequence of films (arterial, capillary, and venous) to evaluate diagnostic findings properly.

Gastrointestinal Bleeding

It has been shown experimentally that angiography can detect bleeding into the GI tract at rates of 0.3 to 1.0 mL per minute or greater. The most common sites of upper GI bleeding are in the stomach and duodenum; therefore, good opacification of the vessels supplying these regions—including the left gastric, gastroduodenal, gastroepiploics, and splenic arteries, and the upper branches of the superior mesenteric artery that supply the duodenum—is imperative. A site of extravasation is sought which appears as a "puddle" or a dense smudge of contrast material that persists after the normal vascular structures are no longer opacified. If the quantity is large enough, this extravasated contrast material may outline the mucosal pattern of the gastric or duodenal lumen (Figs. 4.4, 4.5). Often it is easier to find the bleeding site by first examining late-phase films, looking for a persistent collection of contrast material; if one is found, it can be traced back through earlier phases in order to determine which artery is the source.

Extravasation can be mimicked by dense mucosal staining due to hyperemic mucosa, or to a wedged catheter position with overinjection of contrast material. Generally, close inspection of the films will clarify the situation. Another possible pitfall is mistaking the blush of a normal adrenal gland for a site of extravasation (Fig. 4.6). The key to avoiding this error is to note the characteristic shape and location of the adrenal stain. Processes that cause diffuse bleeding, such as hemorrhagic gastritis, usually will not show discrete areas of extravasation, but may demonstrate marked mucosal hyperemia.

Venous bleeding from esophageal or gastric varices will not be definitively shown by celiac angiography. It can be suggested, however, when the arterial phase does not show a bleeding site, but venous-phase films reveal evidence of portal hypertension, such as varices or hepatofugal flow (Fig. 4.7).

Lower GI bleeding (distal to the duodenum) is difficult to monitor clinically because there is no diagnostic procedure for the area equivalent to passing a nasogastric (NG) tube. The nature of the bleeding may range from melena to bright red blood per rectum. While the appearance of the blood may provide a clue to the level of the bleeding site, it is also largely dependent on the rate of bleeding. Thus an angiographic study for lower GI bleeding should include not only the inferior and superior mesenteric arteries, but the celiac axis as well, as bleeding from a duodenal source can mimic lower GI bleeding. Profuse lower GI bleeding is associated most often with colonic diverticuli. Other causes include AVMs, or angiodysplasia, ulceration, Meckel's diverticulum, ischemia, and, occasionally, tumors. A diverticular source can be suggested specifically when the extravasated contrast material remains in a sharply defined rounded collection on late films, reflecting puddling in the diverticulum itself (Fig. 4.8).

Angiodysplasias are small submucosal vascular malformations that occur in the colon, most often in the cecum. They tend to occur in older patients who may have a history of repeated episodic hemorrhage, or slow continuous GI blood loss. The etiology of colonic angiodysplasia is unclear; there seems to be an association with aortic valve disease and in conditions with poor cardiac output. Angiographically, the lesions usually appear as a small tangle of abnormal arteries with shunting into mesenteric veins; often the easiest way to spot them is to look for these early-draining veins first (Fig. 4.9). In many cases these malformations are multiple; the entire lower GI tract should be studied if one lesion is found. Due to their small size and submucosal location, angiodysplasias may be almost invisible at surgery, and special preparation of the specimen is necessary to find them pathologically.

Transcatheter therapy has a major role in the management of GI bleeding. One approach consists of infusing a vasoconstrictor, such as vasopressin, directly into the vessels shown to be the source of bleeding (see Fig. 4.8b). While this method for the containment of bleeding can be quite effective, the catheter must remain in place for hours or days. This can result in a considerable management problem. This technique will not be effective if the bleeding vessels are incapable of vasoconstriction, as in some inflammatory and neoplastic conditions. The use of vasoconstricting drugs may be contraindicated in patients with severe coronary artery disease. An alternative is transcatheter embolization: A device or substance is inserted through the catheter to occlude the bleeding vessel (see Fig. 4.4c). This has the advantage of producing immediate hemostasis, avoiding the need for an in-dwelling catheter. The extensive collateral circulation of the upper GI tract minimizes the risk of tissue ischemia following embolization.

Embolization and infusion of vasoconstrictors are used in the management of lower GI bleeding as well, but the risk of ischemia after embolization is significantly higher than in the upper GI tract, owing to the much poorer collateral supply.

Lesions Impairing Visceral Flow

Impaired blood flow in the visceral circulation may be acute or chronic. When acute, the results are catastrophic if diagnosis and treatment are not carried out within hours of the onset of symptoms. Chronic visceral occlusive disease is tolerated fairly well by most patients, many of whom present with nonspecific abdominal complaints of many years' duration.

Acute intestinal ischemia is usually caused by an arterial embolus, usually of cardiac origin (Fig. 4.10). Patients typically present with acute abdominal pain and tenderness, bloody diarrhea, and abdominal distension due to ileus. If there is a history of cardiac arrhythmia, embolus should be suspected and emergency angiography performed. Biplane aortography first visualizes the origins of the visceral trunks in the lateral view prior to selective catheterization, which might cause a proximal embolus to fragment and shower more distally.

Acute ischemia also may be seen in patients with severely compromised cardiac output ("low-flow state"), or intense vasoconstriction due to other causes. This entity is referred to as "nonocclusive mesenteric ischemia", and may show a characteristic appearance of diffusely narrowed and beaded mesenteric branches. In addition to correcting the low-flow state, infusion of vasodilators directly into a catheter in the superior mesenteric artery may result in marked clinical improvement.

Patients with severe atherosclerosis often have involvement of the proximal visceral trunks. Since the involvement is a gradual process, there is time for collateral circulation to develop (Fig. 4.11). We have encountered asymptomatic patients in whom the celiac and superior mesenteric origins were completely occluded, and the visceral circulation was supplied only by a hypertrophied inferior mesenteric artery (Fig. 4.12). Obviously, a patient whose entire GI tract is being supplied by only one of these trunks will suffer disastrous intestinal ischemia if that trunk occludes.

"Celiac axis compression syndrome" is a controversial entity that is described most often in young, thin female patients who complain of upper abdominal pain and diarrhea following meals. The symptoms may be so distressing that considerable weight loss occurs. On physical examination, an upper abdominal bruit is audible, and angiography shows a marked extrinsic impression on the superior aspect of the main celiac trunk (Fig. 4.13). This is due to a crossing diaphragmatic ligament, which can be released surgically without much difficulty. The controversy surrounding this syndrome concerns whether the symptoms are in fact due to the arterial narrowing, although many patients do report relief of symptoms after surgery.

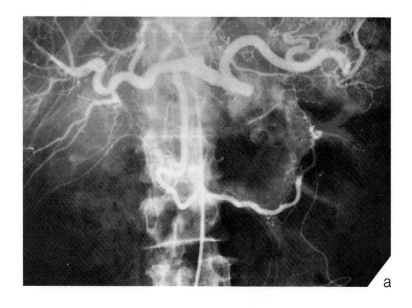

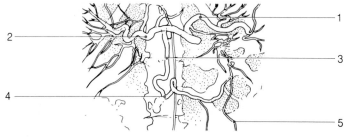

1 Splenic artery	6 Liver
2 Hepatic artery	7 Spleen
3 Gastroduodenal artery	8 Splenic vein
4 Gastroepiploic artery	9 Portal vein
5 Omental vessel	10 Intrahepatic portal circulation

Fig. 4.1 Normal celiac axis arteriogram. *a An arterial-phase film from a selective celiac axis injection. The examination demonstrates the splenic, hepatic, gastroduodenal, and the gastroepiploic arteries as well as branches of these vessels. Small omental vessels are demonstrated also. b A mucosal-phase film from the same injection demonstrates dif-*

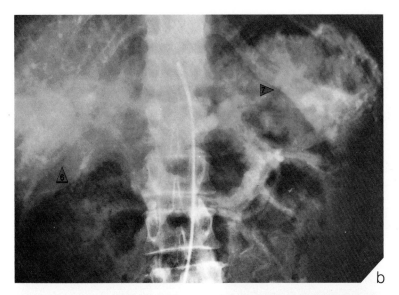

b

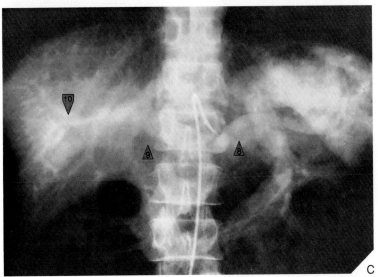

c

fuse opacification of the liver (arrow 6) *and spleen parenchyma (arrow 7)*
as well as a mucosal blush over the stomach. **c** *The late phase, or portal*
phase, of the same injection demonstrates opacification of the splenic
vein (arrow 8), *portal vein* (arrow 9), *and intrahepatic portal circulation*
(arrow 10).

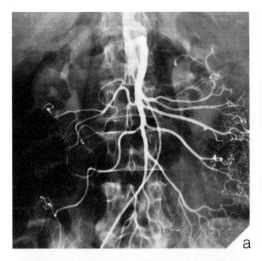 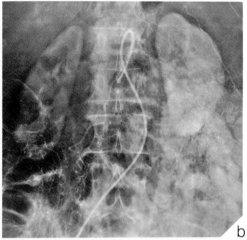

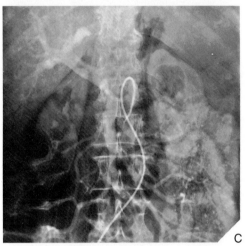

Fig. 4.2 Normal superior mesenteric arteriogram. *a An arterial-phase film from a selective study of the superior mesenteric artery demonstrates this vessel which originates anteriorly from the abdominal aorta at the level of the T12–L1 disc space. This vessel supplies the duodenum, jejunum, ileum, and the proximal colon. b A capillary-phase film from the superior mesenteric artery injection demonstrates the normal diffuse mucosal blush of the small intestine. c The venous-phase film demonstrates opacification of the branch mesenteric, the superior mesenteric, and the main portal veins.*

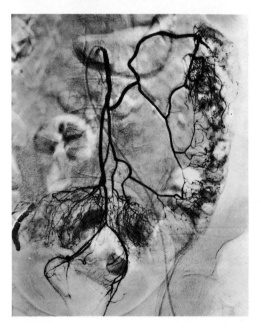

Fig. 4.3 Normal inferior mesenteric arteriogram. *A selective study of the inferior mesenteric artery, which generally originates anteriorly and slightly directed to the left at the L3–4 disc space level. This is a subtraction film, which shows the arterial branching more clearly. The rectum is supplied both by the inferior mesenteric artery and by branches of the hypogastric arteries.*

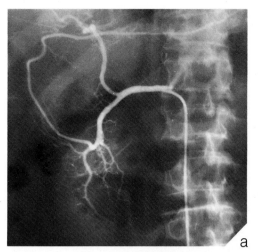

Fig. 4.4 Duodenal hemorrhage. *a* A 76-year-old man presented with massive upper GI bleeding suspected to be of duodenal origin. An early film of a selective injection into the gastroduodenal artery demonstrates the normal appearance of the duodenal branches. *b* The later-phase film of the same injection shows a small smudge of contrast material (arrow) *in the region of the duodenum, which represents the site of bleeding.* *c* *Transcatheter therapy was used to manage this hemorrhage. Several stainless steel coils (arrow)* were inserted through the catheter to occlude the gastroduodenal artery. This follow-up arteriogram shows no further filling of the midportion of the gastroduodenal artery, and no further extravasation. The bleeding stopped promptly. Generally this type of embolization in the upper GI tract is quite safe due to the rich collateral blood supply of the upper abdominal organs.

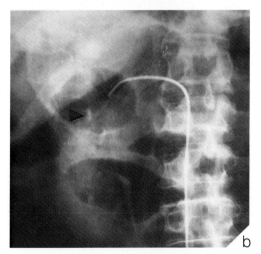

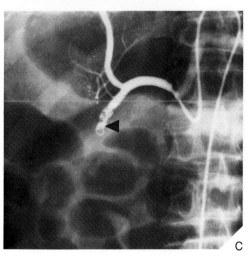

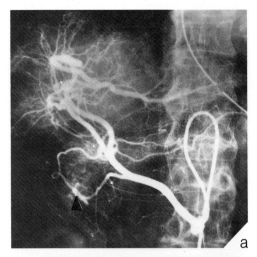

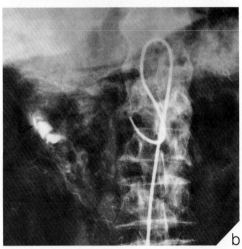

Fig. 4.5 Duodenal hemorrhage. *A patient presented with massive upper GI bleeding of duodenal origin.* **a** *The arterial-phase film demonstrates an irregular collection of contrast material beginning to appear next to one of the duodenal branches (arrow).* **b** *The later-phase film demonstrates a large puddle of extravasated contrast material outlining the mucosal pattern of the duodenum (arrow).*

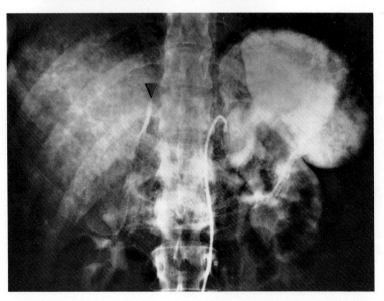

Fig. 4.6 Adrenal blush mimicking a hemorrhage. *A mucosal-phase film from a celiac study of a patient admitted for upper GI bleeding demonstrates an elongated triangular stain (arrow) to the right of the T12 vertebral body. The shape and location of this stain are characteristic for the normal blush of the adrenal gland, and should not be confused with a site of extravasation.*

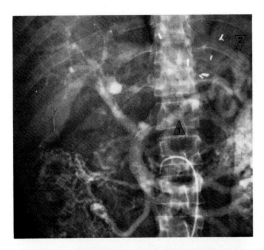

Fig. 4.7 Gastric varices. *A 47-year-old alcoholic patient presented with massive upper GI bleeding. The celiac and superior mesenteric study showed no evidence of active arterial extravasation, but the venous-phase films demonstrated evidence of severe portal hypertension. This is a venous-phase film from the superior mesenteric injection, demonstrating hepatofugal flow into the splenic vein (arrow 1) as well as filling of gastric varices (arrow 2). In this type of situation, the findings are strongly suggestive of a venous source of bleeding.*

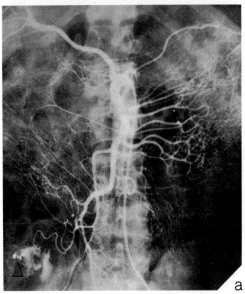

a

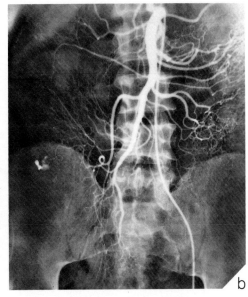

b

Fig. 4.8 Bleeding colonic diverticulum.
a This is a superior mesenteric arteriogram of a 59-year-old patient with massive lower GI bleeding. The examination demonstrates gross extravasation of contrast in the cecum (arrow). The primary point of extravasation is a sharply defined rounded collection of contrast, which represents a diverticulum. In this case, an

attempt was made to control the bleeding by infusing vasopressin directly into the catheter in the superior mesenteric artery. b A follow-up film demonstrates diffuse vasoconstriction and a considerably reduced amount of extravasation in the cecum, although some puddling remains.

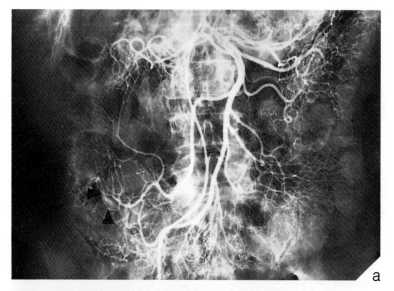

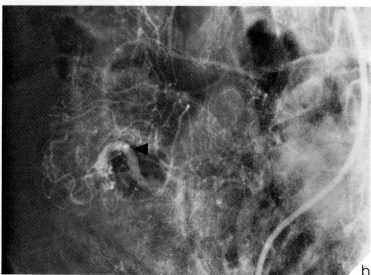

Fig. 4.9 Angiodysplasia of the cecum. *a Superior mesenteric arteriogram of a 66-year-old man with chronic congestive failure and recurrent episodes of massive lower GI bleeding demonstrates a subtle abnormality in the region of the cecum. If this region is examined closely, an early draining vein can be seen (arrows).* **b** *A magnified view of this area in a slightly later phase shows more clearly this early draining vein (arrow). The findings are characteristic of colonic angiodysplasia, a specific type of vascular malformation. These are most often found in the cecum, although they may be located anywhere in the colon, and may be multiple.*

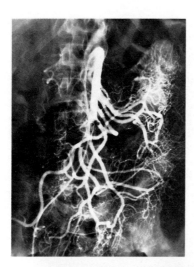

Fig. 4.10 Acute superior mesenteric artery embolus. *A 76-year-old man presented with acute abdominal pain and diarrhea after aortic valve replacement and cardioversion for atrial fibrillation. The superior mesenteric arteriogram shows a large filling defect within the superior mesenteric artery (arrow), extending into several branches. The findings are typical of an acute embolus. When embolization to the visceral circulation is suspected, the initial study should be a biplane aortogram to rule out the presence of emboli at the origins of the vessels, which could shower more distally during catheterization.*

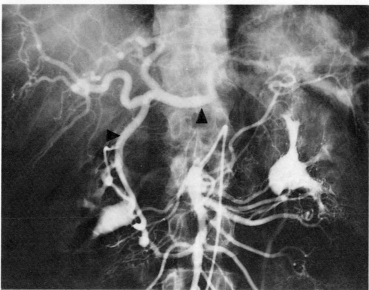

Fig. 4.11 Chronic occlusion of celiac axis. *A superior mesenteric artery injection demonstrates filling of the celiac axis (arrow 1) through the gastroduodenal collateral pathway (arrow 2). This type of filling is seen when there is a high-grade stenosis or complete occlusion of the proximal celiac trunk. Due to good collateral reconstitution, this type of occlusive process is often asymptomatic.*

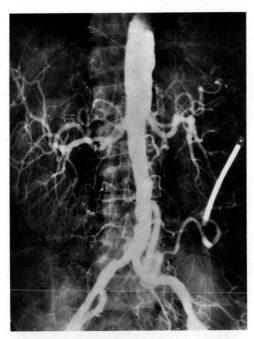

Fig. 4.12 Chronic occlusion of celiac axis and superior mesenteric artery. *Aortogram of a 58-year-old woman with diffuse atherosclerosis and complaints of abdominal pain after eating. The film demonstrates poor filling of the celiac axis, no filling of the superior mesenteric artery, and filling of a hypertrophied inferior mesenteric trunk (arrow). The entire visceral circulation can be carried by any one of these three visceral trunks if the process develops slowly, and adequate collateral pathways develop.*

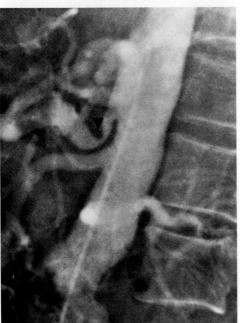

Fig. 4.13 Celiac axis compression syndrome. *A lateral view of a flush aortogram demonstrates the origins of the celiac and superior mesenteric arteries. The proximal celiac trunk shows a sharp impression on its superior margin (arrow), with post-stenotic dilation. This finding is characteristic of celiac axis compression due to a crossing diaphragmatic ligament. The relationship of this finding to upper abdominal symptomatology is controversial.*

ABDOMINAL TUMORS

Tumors of the abdominal organs vary widely in angiographic appearance. Some lesions are detectable by their abnormal internal vasculature; these abnormal arteries are referred to as "tumor vessels" or "neovascularity." Tumor vessels may have a bizarre appearance, with failure to taper normally, sharp angulations, contrast puddling or staining, and, in some cases, arteriovenous shunting. Some tumors, particularly pancreatic carcinoma, show no significant intrinsic vascularity, but are demonstrable by their effect on arteries and veins in the region (encasement). The degree of vascularity does not denote whether the tumor is benign or malignant, but certain patterns are characteristic and will be discussed in the sections on individual abdominal organs.

Liver: Benign and Malignant Tumors

Benign lesions that are commonly encountered in the liver include cysts, cavernous hemangiomas, focal nodular hyperplasia, and hepatic adenomas. Cysts are not true neoplasms, and are rarely of clinical significance (Fig. 4.14); the widespread use of CT and ultrasound has shown them to be much more common than previously thought. Cavernous hemangiomas are the most common benign neoplasm of the liver. Rarely symptomatic unless they bleed or rupture, they generally do not require specific therapy. The diagnosis can nearly always be confirmed by CT, but the angiographic appearance is characteristic (Fig. 4.15). Focal nodular hyperplasia is a benign hamartomatous lesion composed of normal liver tissue, fibrous septae, and numerous blood vessels. These lesions are generally asymptomatic, most often encountered in young women, and may be single or multiple (Fig. 4.16). Hepatic adenomas are benign neoplasms; they may bleed spontaneously, sometimes presenting as a free intraabdominal hemorrhage. There is an increased incidence of these lesions in women who have taken oral contraceptives. Unlike focal nodular hyperplasia, these lesions are usually solitary, and may be extremely large (Fig. 4.17). Pathologically, they are composed of hepatocytes, but show no bile ducts or Kupffer cells. Unlike focal nodular hyperplasia, these lesions never show uptake on radiocolloid liver scans, due to the absence of Kupffer cells.

Metastatic disease is the most frequently encountered malignant process in the liver. The lesions may be single, but are more often multiple, a finding that strongly suggests the diagnosis. The blood supply of normal hepatic parenchyma is principally derived from the portal circulation; metastatic lesions and most primary malignant liver tumors are supplied by the hepatic arterial circulation. Metastatic lesions vary in angiographic appearance; their degree of vascularity is largely determined by the type of primary tumor (Figs. 4.18, 4.19).

Primary liver tumors (hepatomas) are variable in their angiographic appearance also, but tend to be large and hypervascular, often showing marked hypertrophy of the feeding arteries. A distinctive finding that is highly suggestive of this diagnosis is shunting from the hepatic arteries to the portal veins (arterioportal shunting) (Figs. 4.20, 4.21). This shunting may result in portal hypertension.

Spleen

The spleen may be affected by trauma, infection, tumor, or infarction. All of these conditions are more appropriately studied by CT or ultrasound than by angiography, at least initially. Angiographically the normal spleen appears as a rounded triangular organ, tucked under the diaphragm in the left upper quadrant. The splenic artery is frequently tortuous, quite commonly showing atherosclerotic calcification in older patients, as well as occasional aneurysm formation (Fig. 4.22).

The venous phase of the splenic arteriogram shows opacification of the splenic vein, which is part of the portal system. The splenic vein is large, and its course is straight, unlike the undulating splenic artery. Since the splenic vein is in intimate contact with the pancreas, it is often affected by abnormalities in this organ, particularly inflammation or neoplasm.

Splenic rupture can be diagnosed by angiography (formerly the "gold standard"), but lobulation and other normal variants in the configuration of the spleen can lead to errors (both false positive and false negative).

The spleen may be involved by primary or metastatic neoplasms as well as diffusely infiltrated in leukemias or lymphomas. The angiographic findings tend to be nonspecific; however, masses, splenic enlargement, or stretching of intrasplenic vessels may be seen.

Pancreas

Until fairly recently, angiography was one of the only techniques available for imaging the pancreas. Other imaging modalities have largely replaced angiography, but it remains a useful technique for delineating regional vascular anatomy and determining potential resectability of pancreatic carcinoma prior to surgery.

The pancreas receives its blood supply from the celiac axis and superior mesenteric arteries. The head of the gland is supplied by the pancreaticoduodenal arteries, which originate from both the gastroduodenal (a celiac branch) and the superior mesenteric arteries (Fig. 4.23). The body of the pancreas is supplied by the dorsal pancreatic artery, a small vessel which usually originates from the inferior aspect of the celiac axis itself. Several small arteries, which supply the distal body and tail of the pancreas, arise distally from the splenic artery. The largest of these branches is termed the pancreatic magna. All three of these sources contribute to form the transverse pancreatic artery, which runs through the middle of the gland (Fig. 4.24).

Adenocarcinoma, the most common malignant pancreatic tumor, is almost always hypovascular or avascular on angiography. Adeno-carcinoma is detected by its effect on normal vessels in the pancreas and the surrounding region. The angiographic term for this effect is "encasement", referring to tubular narrowing, loss of normal tapering, abrupt angulation, and sometimes complete occlusion (Figs. 4.25, 4.26a). The vessels involved depend on the size and location of the tumor within the pancreas, and may include intrapancreatic, gastroduodenal, splenic, and common hepatic arteries, superior mesenteric branches, and sometimes the main celiac or superior mesenteric trunks themselves. Tumor encasement must be distinguished from atherosclerotic or inflammatory involvement, which can have a similar appearance. Inflammation, particularly pancreatitis, can produce vascular abnormalities that resemble the changes seen with neoplasm, and differentiation may not always be possible.

The portal venous phase is probably the most important part of the radiologic examination if carcinoma of the pancreas is suspected. The splenic and proximal superior mesenteric veins have an intimate anatomical relationship to the pancreas. Because veins are more compressible than arteries, angiograms usually show abnormalities of the veins (e.g., compression by the tumor) before any arterial abnormalities are apparent. Venous involvement ranges from encasement to complete occlusion, and is commonly seen in advanced lesions (Figs. 4.25b, 4.26b).

Other tumors that occur in the pancreas include islet cell tumors, which may or may not be endocrinologically active, cystadenomas, cystadenocarcinomas, and metastatic disease (Figs. 4.27, 4.28).

Stomach, Small and Large Intestine

There are more effective and less invasive means of diagnosing most neoplasms of the GI tract than angiography, so it is seldom used for this purpose. One situation in which it may be useful, though, is the investigation of occult GI bleeding. Ulceration of submucosal tumors in the stomach or small bowel may be extremely difficult to detect on barium studies, CT, or endoscopy. Leiomyomas in particular are often quite vascular, and may be associated with massive intermittent GI bleeding (Fig. 4.29).

Angiodysplasias of the colon are malformations rather than neoplasms and are discussed in the section on gastrointestinal bleeding, earlier in this chapter.

Kidneys

The most common mass encountered in the kidney is the simple cyst, a benign lesion usually discovered incidentally. Ultrasound is the best study to confirm the diagnosis, but the angiographic findings are also distinctive (Fig. 4.30).

Benign solid neoplasms of the kidney, which include adenomas, onocytomas, and angiomyolipomas, are relatively rare, and may be difficult or impossible to distinguish angiographically from renal cancer, although certain features are suggestive (Figs. 4.31, 4.32).

Hypernephroma, or renal cell carcinoma, is the most frequent malignant tumor of the kidney. Most of these tumors have a characteristic angiographic appearance consisting of enlarged feeding arteries, marked hypervascularity, arteriovenous shunting, and, in some cases, extension of tumor into the renal vein and inferior vena cava (Figs. 4.33, 4.34). These lesions may be very large, with flow so rapid that two or three times the normal contrast injection rate and volume is required for adequate opacification. Since renal vein involvement is common, the venous phase must be evaluated carefully and, if there is any question, direct study of the inferior vena cava and renal vein should be performed. Some hypernephromas are hypovascular or almost entirely avascular, and may contain a cystic component.

Transitional cell carcinoma is generally hypovascular on angiography but arteries in the region of the tumor may show evidence of spreading, infiltration, or encasement (Fig. 4.35).

Adrenal Glands

With a few exceptions, CT and ultrasound have replaced angiography as the imaging modality of choice in the diagnosis of adrenal disease. The adrenal glands receive their blood supply from three sources: the renal artery, the aorta, and the inferior phrenic artery. The small caliber of the adrenal branches, and the need to inject all of them to completely evaluate the gland, results in a prolonged, tedious examination (Fig. 4.36).

In the past, adrenal venography has been used to investigate adrenal abnormalities (Fig. 4.37). The technique offers the advantage of obtaining adrenal vein samples that are diagnostic in many hormone-secreting adrenal tumors. A distinct risk of adrenal venography is rupture of the capsule of the gland, which may result in irreversible ablation of function. This has also been done intentionally in some conditions to produce a nonsurgical adrenalectomy.

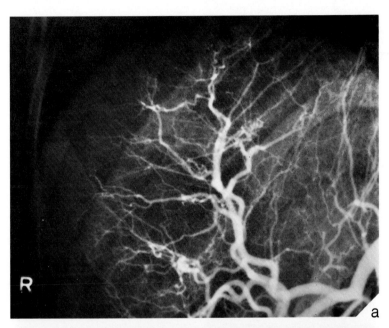

a

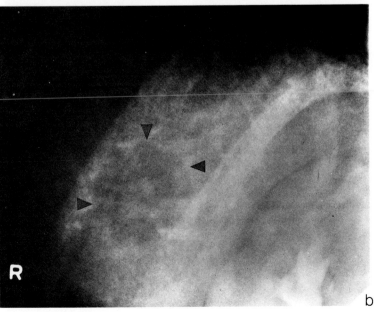

b

Fig. 4.14 Liver cyst. A defect in the right lobe of the liver was seen on a liver-spleen scan in a 35-year-old woman with a history of lymphoma. (This case occurred before the era of computed tomography.) **a** The arterial phase demonstrates minimal stretching of the intrahepatic arteries, with no evidence of abnormal vascularity. **b** The hepatogram, or parenchymal phase of the study, shows a sharply marginated round avascular area (arrows). These findings are compatible with a simple cyst of the liver.

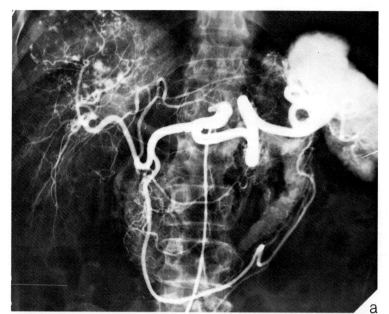

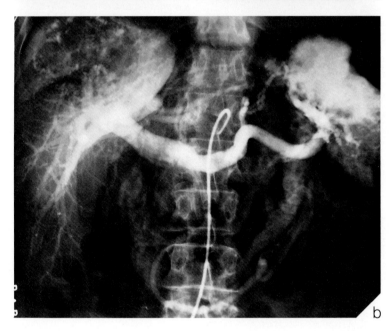

Fig. 4.15 Cavernous hemangioma. *A 70-year-old woman was found to have a large mass in the right lobe of the liver on sonography and computed tomography.*
a The celiac axis injection demonstrates numerous small puddles of contrast on the periphery of the lesion. b The late phase of the examination shows opacification of the portal system with persistent dense puddling of contrast in the right lobe lesion. Such puddling with prolonged stasis is quite characteristic for benign cavernous hemangioma. This type of lesion is generally asymptomatic and requires no specific therapy.

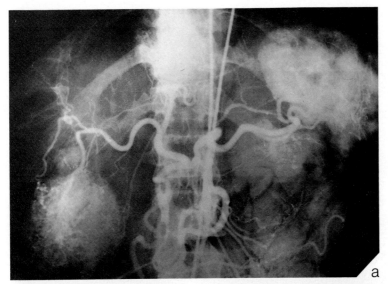

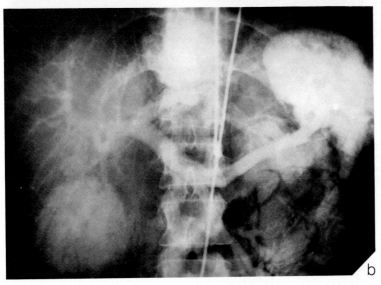

Fig. 4.16 Focal nodular hyperplasia. *Computed tomography and ultrasonography demonstrated a mass in the right lobe of the liver in this 38-year-old woman who was admitted complaining of dull right upper quadrant pain.* ***a*** *The arteriogram demonstrates a large round hypervascular mass extending from the inferior aspect of the right lobe. There is an enlarged feeding artery and a faint radiating vascular pattern is seen within the mass. No arteriovenous shunting is present. Also note the presence of a common origin of the celiac and superior mesenteric arteries, a normal variant.* ***b*** *The late phase of the same injection demonstrates good opacification of the portal system and dense staining of the rounded liver lesion. These findings are quite consistent with focal nodular hyperplasia, a benign hamartomatous lesion.*

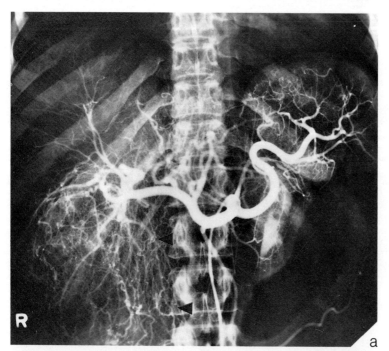

Fig. 4.17 Hepatic adenoma.
a Hepatic adenomas, like focal nodular hyperplasia, are usually encountered in young women. Hepatic adenomas may bleed spontaneously, as occurred in this 28-year-old woman who presented with free intraabdominal hemorrhage. The celiac axis injection demonstrates a large hypervascular mass involving the inferior aspect of the right lobe of the liver (arrows). Numerous bizarre blood vessels are noted within the mass, with no discernible organized pattern. *b* A late-phase film demonstrates the large hypervascular mass, with a defect in its inferior margin most likely representing the area of hemorrhage. These lesions have been associated with oral contraceptive intake.

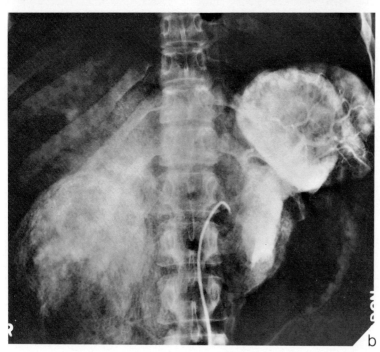

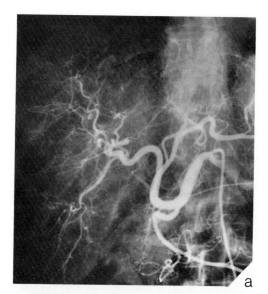

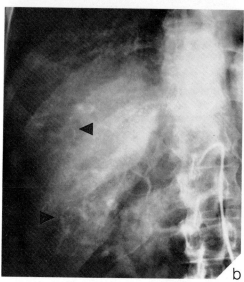

Fig. 4.18 Hypovascular hepatic metastases.
A 62-year-old woman with a history of colon resection for carcinoma presented with a rising carcinoembryonic antigen (CEA) titer. Computed tomography showed some inhomogeneity, but no definite lesions. **a** *Arterial phase of the celiac arteriogram shows no significant abnormality.* **b** *The hepatogram phase, however, demonstrates several round avascular lesions with moderately vascular rims (arrows). This hypovascular type of lesion is commonly associated with metastases of carcinoma of the colon, breast, and lung.*

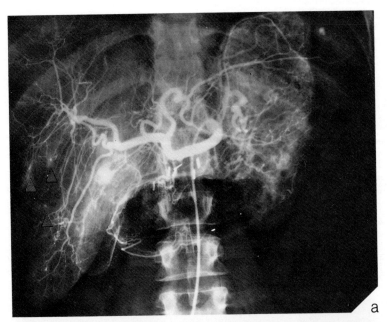

a

Fig. 4.19 Hypervascular hepatic metastases. *This 31-year-old woman, who had undergone a total pancreatectomy for a functioning islet cell tumor 1 year previously, presented with recurrent symptoms. **a** The celiac injection demonstrates multiple hypervascular lesions (arrows) scattered throughout the right lobe of the liver. **b** The late-phase film shows these lesions more clearly. Hypervascular metastatic lesions tend to be associated with hypernephromas, some sarcomas, carcinoid, primary endocrine, and, occasionally, colon carcinomas. The thin-walled curvilinear structure (arrow) overlapping the inferior edge of the right lobe of the liver represents the blush of the normal gallbladder wall.*

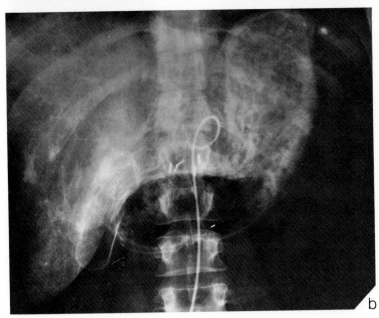

b

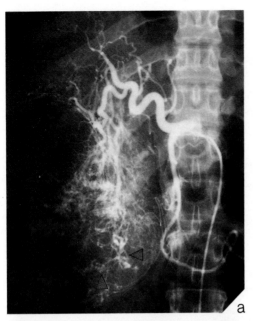

Fig. 4.20 Hepatoma. *A 39-year-old male with a 10-year history of chronic active hepatitis presented with a large abdominal mass.*
***a** Celiac arteriography demonstrated the mass to be of hepatic origin. The bizarre tumor vessels* (arrows) *are quite characteristic of a malignant tumor such as hepatoma. **b** The late-phase film demonstrates filling of intrahepatic portal vein radicles* (arrows). *Portal venous radicles would not normally fill from a hepatic arterial injection, and this type of arterial-portal shunting is quite characteristic of hepatoma.*

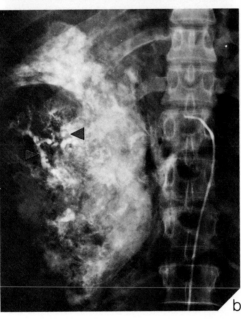

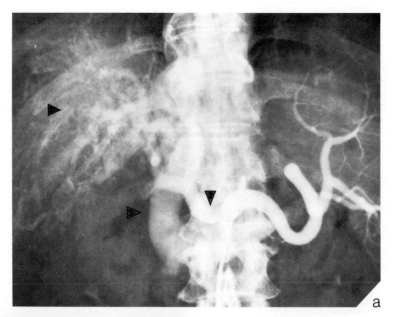

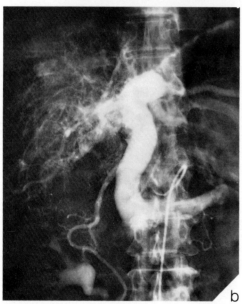

Fig. 4.21 Hepatoma with esophageal varices secondary to arterioportal shunting. *This 72-year-old man presented with massive upper GI bleeding.* **a** *The celiac arteriogram shows a hypervascular mass in the liver (arrow 1). There is massive shunting from the hepatic artery (arrow 2) to the main portal vein (arrow 3).* **b** *The later-phase film shows further filling of the portal vein and hepatofugal flow, which is responsible for the variceal bleeding.*

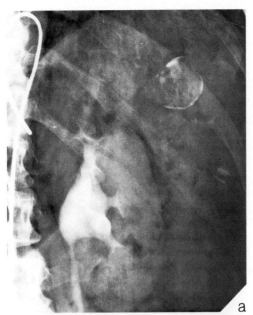

Fig. 4.22 Calcified splenic artery aneurysm.
a When a 45-year-old woman had abdominal films taken to evaluate back pain, a rounded curvilinear calcification was noted incidentally in the left upper quadrant. This type of calcification is quite typical of that seen in blood vessels, particularly aneurysms. **b** A splenic arteriogram demonstrates a large aneurysm in the hilus of the spleen, which corresponds to the area of calcification (arrows).

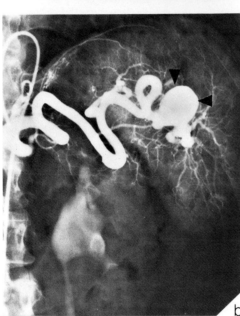

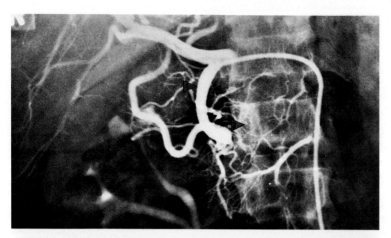

Fig. 4.23 Arterial supply to head of pancreas. *An injection into the gastroduodenal artery* (arrow 1) *demonstrates the normal pancreaticoduodenal arteries that supply the head of the pancreas* (arrow 2). *The superior mesenteric artery also contributes to this circulation.*

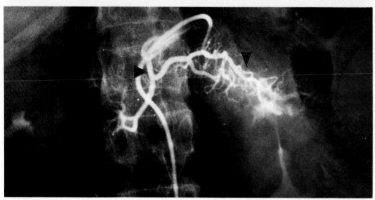

Fig. 4.24 Arterial supply to body and tail of pancreas. *The catheter tip is in the pancreatic magna, a branch of the splenic artery. Injection fills the transverse pancreatic artery* (arrow 1) *and there is retrograde filling of the dorsal pancreatic artery* (arrow 2), *a branch of the main celiac trunk. No abnormalities are seen on this particular study. Angiographically, the pancreas is not a very vascular organ. Often the capillary phase of a good-quality celiac arteriogram will show a faint parenchymal blush of the organ, particularly in the body and tail. The pancreatic head is frequently difficult to distinguish from the mucosal blush of the intimately associated duodenal sweep.*

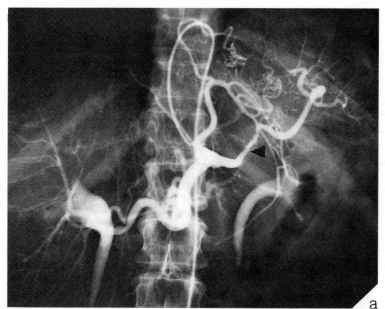

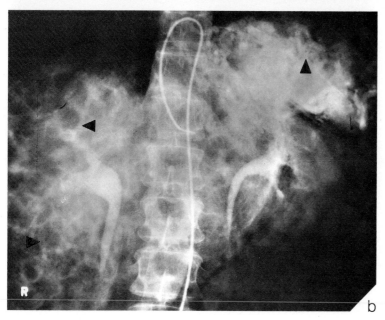

Fig. 4.25 Adenocarcinoma of the pancreas. *a Celiac axis study of a 61-year-old man, who presented with abdominal pain and weight loss. The film demonstrates irregular narrowing of the midportion of the splenic artery (arrow). This type of tubular narrowing is referred to as "encasement," and is characteristic of involvement of blood vessels by a malignant process. **b** The late-phase film does not demonstrate opacification of the splenic vein, which has been completely occluded by the tumor. Collateral vessels may be noted in the region of the spleen (arrow 1). Also visible are numerous hypovascular masses within the liver (arrows 2), representing widespread metastatic liver disease. The findings are classic for pancreatic adenocarcinoma with liver metastasis.*

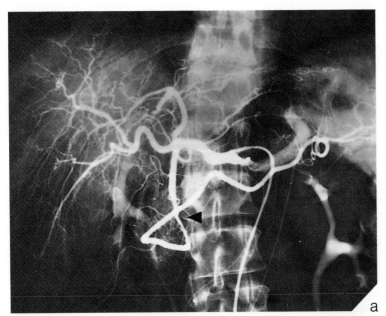

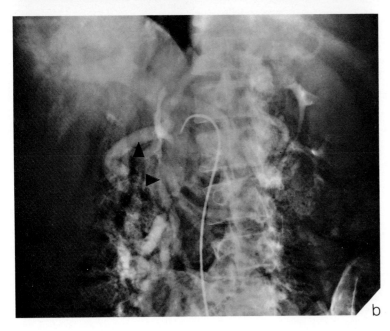

Fig. 4.26 Adenocarcinoma of the pancreas. *This 49-year-old man presented with abdominal pain and weight loss. Computed tomography showed a mass in the uncinate process of the pancreas. Angiography was performed to evaluate the potential for resectability.* **a** *The common hepatic artery injection demonstrates a long narrowed segment of the distal gastroduodenal artery* (arrow), *but no other significant abnormalities.* **b** *The venous phase of the superior mesenteric artery injection demonstrates occlusion of the superior mesenteric vein* (arrow 1), *with filling of collateral venous channels* (arrow 2). *This type of major venous encasement implies the presence of an unresectable tumor.*

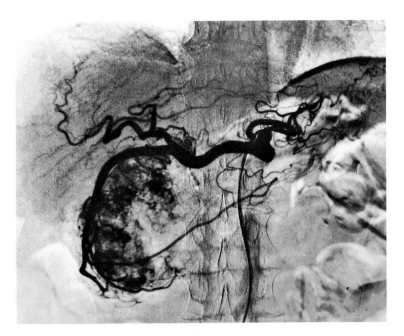

Fig. 4.27 Islet cell tumor of the pancreas. *Islet cell tumors of the pancreas may or may not be endocrinologically active. Tumors that secrete hormone actively tend to be diagnosed when quite small, due to the severe clinical symptomatology. Nonfunctioning islet cell tumors often reach a large size before being detected. In this case, the patient presented with a palpable abdominal mass. The arteriogram demonstrates a huge hypervascular mass in the head of the pancreas. The gastroduodenal artery is enlarged, and it is draped around the mass. Islet cell tumors, whether functioning or nonfunctioning, tend to be hypervascular.*

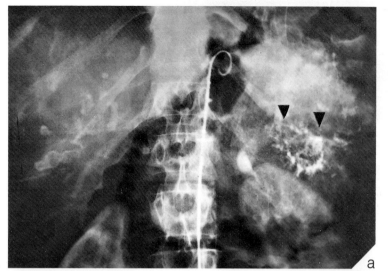

Fig. 4.28 Cystadenoma–cystadenocarcinoma of the pancreas. *Cystadenomas and cystadenocarcinomas frequently reach a large size before clinical detection. As their names imply, both contain cystic and solid elements, and both frequently show internal calcification, often in a stellate pattern (**a**, arrows). The tumor is typically hypervascular, as shown in **b** and in **c**, which demonstrate hypertrophied pancreatic branches (arrows) of the splenic artery feeding the lesion in the tail of the pancreas; **c** also shows compression of the splenic vein (arrow).*

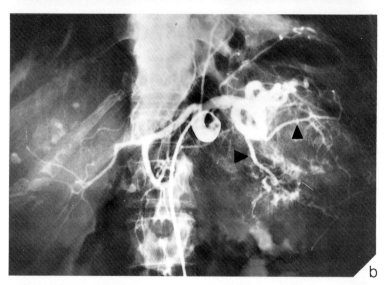

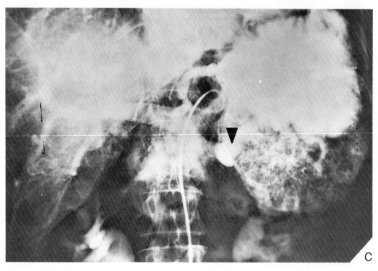

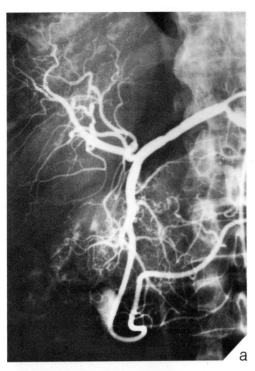

a

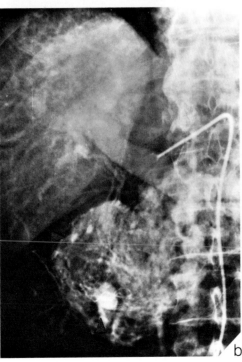

b

Fig. 4.29 Gastric leiomyoma. *This patient presented with intermittent upper GI bleeding and negative endoscopy.* **a** *The common hepatic injection demonstrates a large hypervascular mass supplied by gastroduodenal branches.* **b** *The late-phase film shows fairly dense staining (arrows). At surgery, this lesion was found to be a gastric leiomyoma. These lesions may involve the stomach or the small intestine; when they ulcerate, they can be the cause of intermittent massive GI bleeding.*

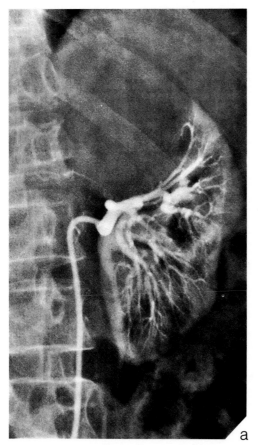
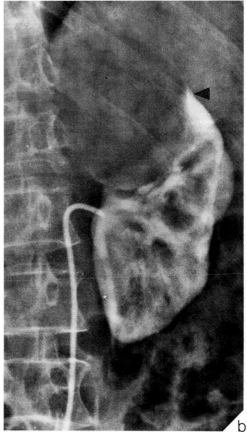

Fig. 4.30 Renal cyst. *Benign renal cysts are extremely common, and are found routinely on CT and ultrasound examinations performed for other reasons. Angiography would not normally be performed to make the diagnosis; however, this case from the pre-CT era demonstrates the classic angiographic findings. **a** There is a large completely avascular mass involving the upper pole of the kidney, displacing the normal intrarenal vessels. **b** The nephrogram phase shows the so-called beak sign at the point where the cyst meets the edge of the renal cortex (arrow).*

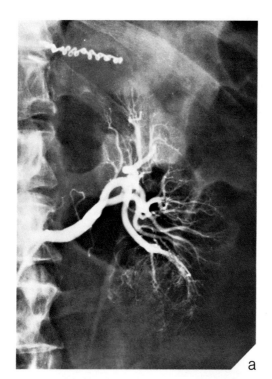

Fig. 4.31 Renal oncocytoma. *Oncocytomas are benign renal parenchymal lesions that are often indistinguishable from hypernephromas prior to surgery. Features that suggest this diagnosis include a sharply marginated round shape, a relatively uniform consistency and, in many cases, the stellate pattern of vessels within the lesion.* ***a, b*** *Arterial and capillary phases of renal arteriogram demonstrate a typical oncocytoma involving the lower pole of the left kidney. A heminephrectomy was performed.*

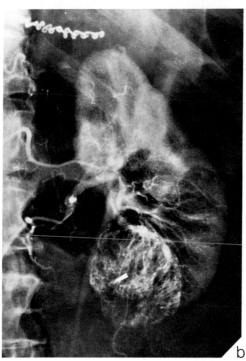

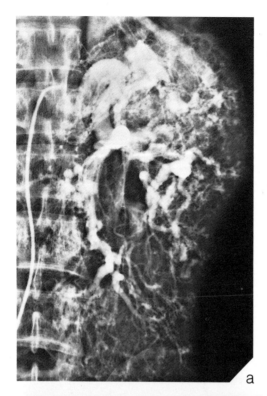

Fig. 4.32 Renal angiomyolipoma. *A 24-year-old man known to have tuberous sclerosis, presented with acute abdominal pain on the left side and a dropping hematocrit.* **a** *The arteriogram demonstrates a huge hypervascular mass involving almost the entire left kidney, with enlarged feeding vessels and pseudoaneurysms, but no evidence of arteriovenous shunting.* **b** *The CT scan shows clearly the large amount of fat within the lesion (arrows), a finding that is pathognomonic for angiomyolipoma, a common lesion in patients with tuberous sclerosis. Though these lesions are benign, they may bleed massively, necessitating nephrectomy.*

a

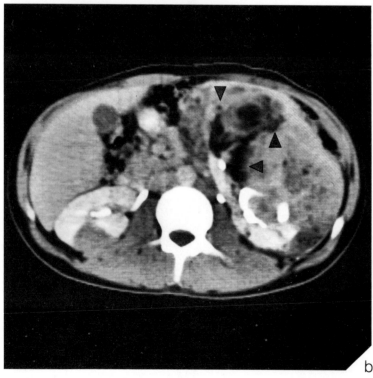

b

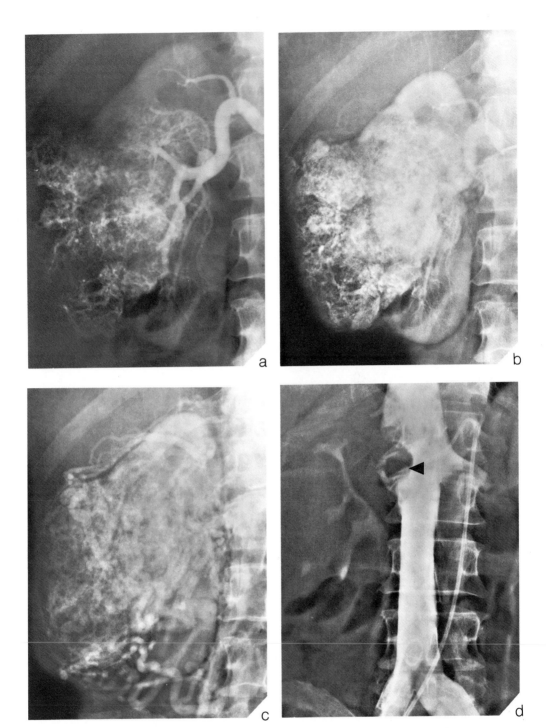

Fig. 4.33 Renal cell carcinoma.
Hypernephroma, or renal cell carcinoma, is the most common malignant tumor of the kidney. In most cases, this lesion has a highly characteristic appearance, as seen in this 58-year-old man who presented with painless gross hematuria. **a, b** *The arteriograms demonstrate a very large, extremely hypervascular mass occupying the midportion of the kidney.* **c** *The late-phase film demonstrates filling of numerous collateral veins, suggesting renal vein obstruction due to tumor invasion.* **d** *This is confirmed by direct inferior venacavography, which shows the tumor thrombus protruding from the right renal vein orifice into the lumen of the cava (arrow). Extension of a tumor into the renal vein is seen commonly, and the tumor thrombus may extend as high as the right atrium.*

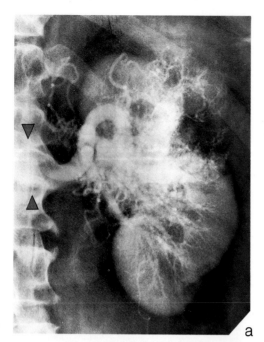

Fig. 4.34 Renal cell carcinoma. *This patient presented with a large hypernephroma involving the left kidney. In this case, there is rapid arteriovenous shunting through the tumor rather than renal vein invasion.* **a** *On the arterial injection, almost immediate opacification of the renal vein (arrows) can be appreciated.* **b** *A later-phase film demonstrates the presence of periureteral collateral veins (arrow), due to the increased venous pressure caused by the arteriovenous shunting.*

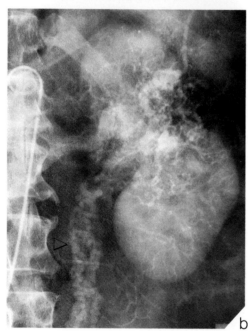

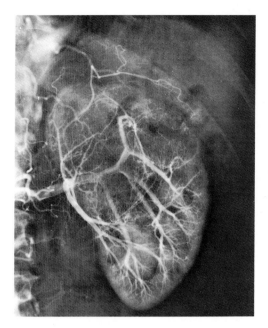

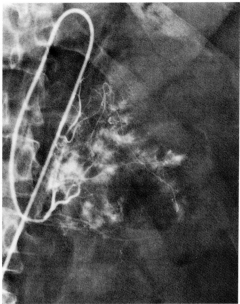

Fig. 4.35 Transitional cell carcinoma. *Unlike renal cell carcinoma, transitional cell carcinoma often appears hypovascular on angiography, as in this 72-year-old man with gross hematuria. The retrograde pyelogram (not shown) showed a large mass filling the left renal pelvis. A hypovascular mass here displaces the blood vessels around the renal pelvis. A fine pattern of neovascularity can be appreciated.*

Fig. 4.36 Adrenal cortical carcinoma. *A selective study of the left inferior adrenal artery in a 46-year-old man with a 3-year history of hypertension and a recent 40-pound weight loss. The study demonstrates a large hypervascular mass involving the adrenal gland. At surgery this was found to be an adrenal cortical carcinoma.*

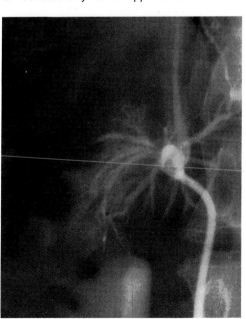

Fig. 4.37 Normal adrenal venogram. *Adrenal venography can be used to evaluate changes in the architecture of a gland as well as to obtain venous samples for evaluating hormone secretion. Adrenal vein sampling is difficult to perform and is somewhat hazardous as overdistension of the veins can result in capsular rupture and loss of glandular function.*

CHAPTER FIVE

*T*he Extremities

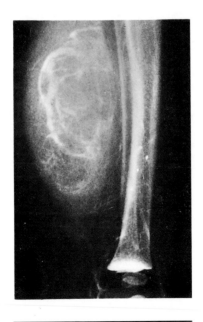

ARTERIOGRAPHY

Modern vascular surgery would not be possible without high-quality angiography, particularly in the extremities. The most common indication is to evaluate atherosclerosis involving the lower extremities, which may present clinically as claudication (cramping on exercise), pain at rest, or actual gangrene. Arteriography is frequently the key to therapeutic decision making and surgical planning. The angiographer should therefore have at least a basic knowledge of vascular surgery to determine precisely what information is required for each particular case. In planning a surgical approach, it is necessary to see not only the actual sites of pathology (stenosis, occlusion, aneurysm, embolus), but the circulation above and below (the inflow and outflow) as well.

Peripheral arteriography is also widely used in the management of suspected vascular trauma. Trauma may result in disruption of vessels with hemorrhage, pseudoaneurysm formation, thrombosis, or extrinsic compression. Early diagnosis and prompt intervention are essential.

Peripheral arteriography is a relatively simple procedure. It carries a low complication rate in experienced hands. The contrast medium injected does result in significant discomfort for the patient, and premedication for pain is given routinely. Digital image processing is a recent development that allows arteriography to be performed with either an intravenous contrast injection or a direct arterial injection of much less concentrated contrast material—in either case there is much less discomfort. It appears likely that in the near future essentially all arteriography will be performed with some type of digital imaging.

Atherosclerotic Disease

Occlusive atherosclerotic disease of the lower extremities is an extremely common clinical problem (Figs. 5.1–5.3). Occlusive disease has a definite predilection for certain sites, one of the earliest of which is the superficial femoral artery at the level of the adductor canal. The pattern of the disease shown in Fig. 5.1 is quite common; it may be associated with severe claudication or frank ischemia. The importance of the deep femoral circulation in preserving limb viability is readily apparent. Femoral–popliteal bypass grafting or percutaneous transluminal angioplasty are used to treat this disorder (Fig. 5.4).

Aneurysmal Disease

In some patients, atherosclerosis is manifested not by narrowing and occlusion of vessels but by abnormal widening of vessels with eventual progression to frank aneurysm formation. Certain sites are prone to this type of disease, including the lower abdominal aorta and the common femoral and popliteal arteries. Often aneurysms in several of these locations coexist in the same patient (Fig. 5.5). Many aneurysms are picked up incidentally on routine physical examination as pulsatile masses. The lesion may be detected because of a complication such as embolization, thrombosis, or rupture (Fig. 5.5).

Figures 5.6–5.8 show how these lesions can be visualized using arteriography; the application of ultrasonography is shown in Fig. 5.9.

Arterial Embolism

Emboli in the peripheral circulation are a common cause of acute ischemia. These emboli may originate from the heart, as in atrial fibrillation associated with mural thrombus (Fig. 5.10); they may also originate from a segment of the peripheral circulation and lodge more distally (Figs. 5.5–5.11). Since these emboli lodge in previously patent vessels, there often is a lack of established collateral blood flow, and ischemia may be severe. In addition to demonstrating the site of embolization, it is obviously essential to investigate the source as well.

Arterial Trauma

Peripheral arteriography is widely used in the management of suspected vascular trauma and has been partly responsible for the steady improvement in limb salvage rates over the past 20 years. Trauma may result in disruption of blood vessels with hemorrhage or pseudoaneurysm formation, intimal tears, thrombosis, or extrinsic compression (Figs. 5.12–5.14). Early diagnosis and prompt intervention are essential. Transcatheter embolization techniques add a new dimension to the management of some of these patients. In many cases, acute hemorrhage can be controlled by injecting embolic materials through the angiographic catheter, obviating surgery.

Tumors

Prior to the era of CT, angiography was commonly performed as a preoperative measure in patients with tumors of the extremities. It is now less commonly used, although the information provided can be extremely helpful in planning resection of the lesion while preserving the maximum amount of normal tissue. Because their angiographic appearance is so variable, it is usually impossible to make a precise diagnosis of tumors in the extremities on this basis. The vascularity may range from being almost entirely absent to profuse (Fig. 5.15). In some instances, the tumor causes encasement of the normal arteries and veins in the region. Embolization through the angiographic catheter has been used in some cases either as a palliative measure or to make extremely vascular lesions more resectable.

Arteriovenous Malformation

Abnormal arteriovenous communications may be congenital or secondary to trauma. The communication may be a simple fistula, allowing shunting from an artery into a vein, or it may consist of an extensive tangle of abnormal arteries and veins, resulting in marked disability and deformity (Figs. 5.16, 5.17). While these lesions are benign by definition, they may be so extensive and progressive that numerous surgical procedures, including amputation, become necessary.

Vasculitis

The arteriographic findings in vasculitis vary widely and depend on the anatomic sites involved as well as the precise nature of the pathologic process. The distal vessels are most often involved, particularly in the hands and feet. The findings may include distal occlusions and irregular stenoses or "beading" (Fig. 5.18). It is important to differentiate fixed narrowing due to vasculitis from transient vascular spasm, which is often seen in arteriography of the hand. The use of intraarterial vasodilators may be necessary to resolve the question.

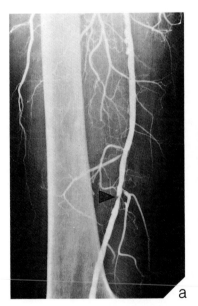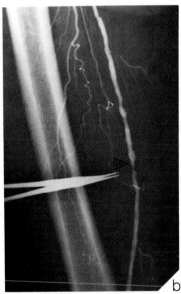

a b

Fig. 5.1 Superficial femoral artery stenosis. *a Atherosclerotic disease begins as a small plaque that progressively impinges on the lumen of the vessel (arrow), in this case, the superficial femoral artery. At this stage of the disease it is unlikely that significant symptomatology will occur. **b** This view demonstrates progression of the atherosclerotic disease to a tight stenosis (arrow). This type of lesion is most often associated with mild claudication on exercise.*

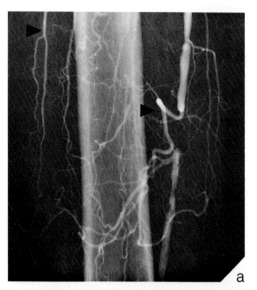

Fig. 5.2 Superficial femoral artery occlusion. *a* Atherosclerosis has progressed to complete occlusion of one segment of the vessel. Note that the vessel is reconstituted by numerous enlarged collateral vessels from the deep femoral circulation (arrow 1) as well as from the termination of the superficial femoral artery (arrow 2). This finding can also be associated with symptoms of exertional pain rather than symptoms at rest. *b* This film of the thighs from a bilateral peripheral arteriogram demonstrates that both superficial femoral arteries are completely occluded. The deep femoral arteries (arrows) are hypertrophied and send collaterals down to the distal thighs. *c* In the same patient, both distal superficial femoral arteries are reconstituted and fill fairly normal-appearing popliteal arteries (arrows).

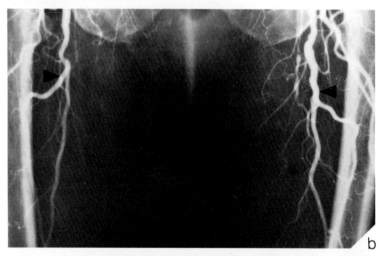

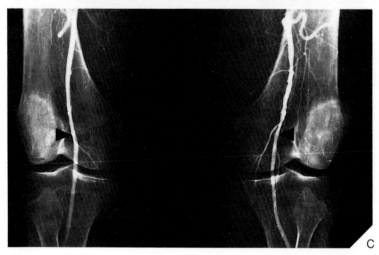

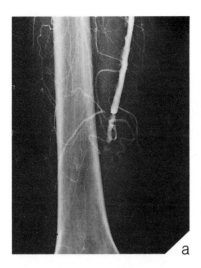 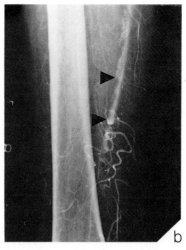

a

b

Fig. 5.3 Acute superficial femoral artery thrombosis. *a Early- and
b late-phase films from a femoral arteriogram in a patient who complained
of intermittent claudication for several years. Two days prior to admission,
he noted an abrupt increase in symptomatology with the onset of rest pain
and loss of some sensation in the foot. Unlike the previous figure in which
well-developed collaterals resupply the distal circulation, the collaterals
are poorly developed in this patient with an acute occlusion of the superficial femoral artery. None of the major trunks distal to the occlusion is
reconstituted. Note some stasis of contrast (arrows) just above the point
of occlusion on the late-phase film, another finding highly suggestive of an
acute process. Such an acute occlusion could represent embolization as
well as thrombosis* in situ. *Because a source of an embolus could not be
found, and because significant atherosclerosis was present in the opposite superficial femoral artery at the same level, this was felt to represent
thrombosis* in situ *secondary to preexisting disease.*

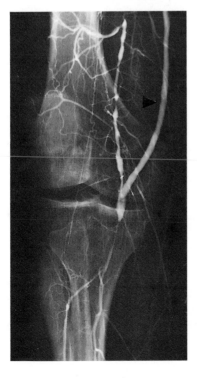

**Fig. 5.4 Femoral artery bypass
graft.** *This is an arteriogram of the
knee region in a patient who underwent a femoral popliteal bypass
graft using a segment of autoge-
nous vein (arrow). While the graft
still remains open, progression of
atherosclerotic disease both above
and below the level of graft insertion is likely to cause graft failure
due to inadequate flow.
Atherosclerosis is a generalized
disorder; bypassing one segment
of the disease does not stop Its
progression.*

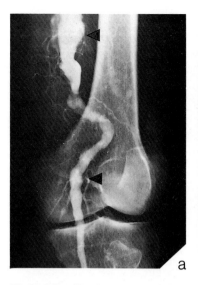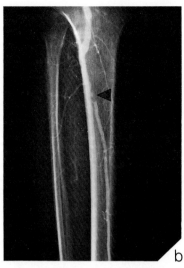

Fig. 5.5 Popliteal artery aneurysm. *a This 71-year-old man was admitted with acute ischemia of the left foot. On physical examination he was found to have a pulsatile mass just above the knee as well as a pulsatile abdominal mass. This film from a femoral arteriogram demonstrates a very irregular fusiform aneurysm of the distal superficial femoral artery (arrow 1) as well as diffuse widening (ectasia) of the popliteal artery (arrow 2). **b** The next lower angiographic field demonstrates complete occlusion of the anterior tibial and peroneal arteries and a radiolucent filling defect within the proximal posterior tibial artery (arrow 3), which is pathognomonic of embolization and presumed to originate from the proximal aneurysm. **c** Popliteal aneurysms are frequently bilateral and, in a very high percentage of cases, are associated with abdominal aortic aneurysms, as was the case with this patient. The abdominal aorta should be evaluated in any patient found to have a popliteal aneurysm.*

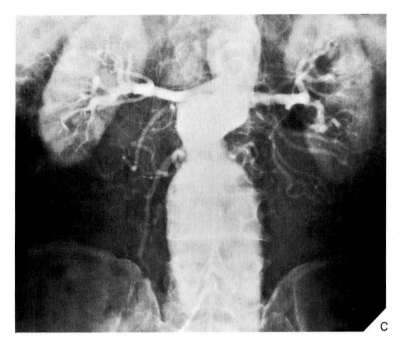

C

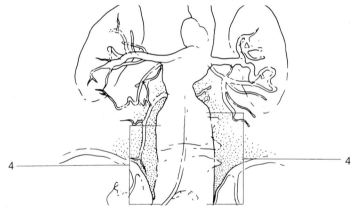

1 Superficial femoral artery aneurysm	3 Filling defect
2 Popliteal artery ectasia	4 Abdominal aortic aneurysm

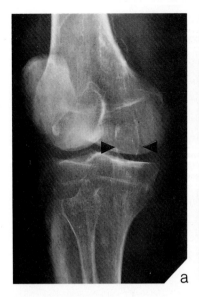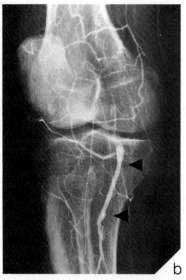

Fig. 5.6 Thrombosis of popliteal artery aneurysm. *a This radiograph demonstrates shell-like calcification of the popliteal artery (arrows) in a patient admitted with acute ischemia of the right lower leg. The increased caliber of the calcified segment suggests the presence of a popliteal aneurysm. **b** The arteriogram demonstrates occlusion of the popliteal artery at the knee with collateral reconstitution of the tibial-peroneal trunk more distally (arrows). This case represents another complication of popliteal aneurysm, namely, spontaneous thrombosis. Since there is often a poorly developed collateral network in these patients, sever ischemia is common when thrombosis occurs.*

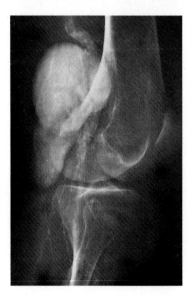

Fig. 5.7 Rupture of popliteal artery aneurysm. *An uncommon complication of popliteal aneurysm is spontaneous rupture. This patient presented with an acutely enlarging mass behind the knee as well as severe ischemia in the lower leg and foot. This late-phase film from a femoral arteriogram demonstrates filling of the popliteal bursa with contrast, representing free rupture of the aneurysm.*

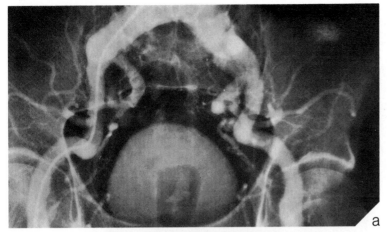

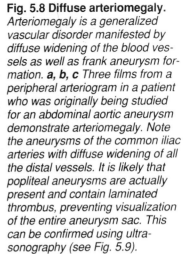

Fig. 5.8 Diffuse arteriomegaly.
Arteriomegaly is a generalized vascular disorder manifested by diffuse widening of the blood vessels as well as frank aneurysm formation. ***a, b, c*** *Three films from a peripheral arteriogram in a patient who was originally being studied for an abdominal aortic aneurysm demonstrate arteriomegaly. Note the aneurysms of the common iliac arteries with diffuse widening of all the distal vessels. It is likely that popliteal aneurysms are actually present and contain laminated thrombus, preventing visualization of the entire aneurysm sac. This can be confirmed using ultrasonography (see Fig. 5.9).*

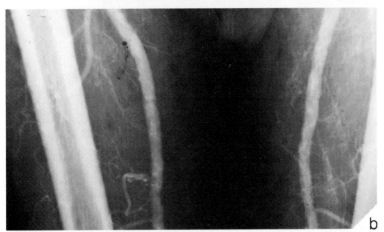

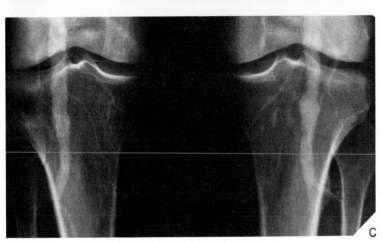

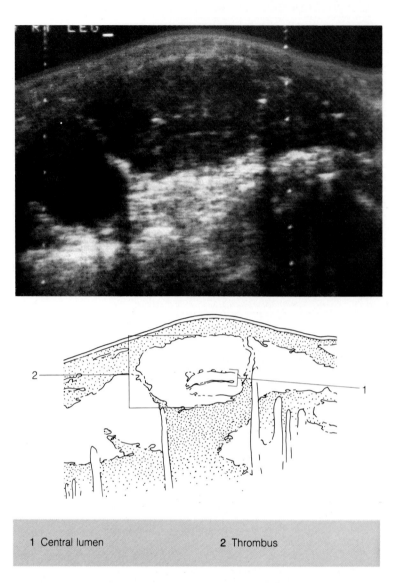

| 1 Central lumen | 2 Thrombus |

Fig. 5.9 Popliteal artery aneurysm. *An ultrasound study of the popliteal region in this patient confirms the presence of an aneurysm. Note the echo-free central lumen and the surrounding thrombus.*

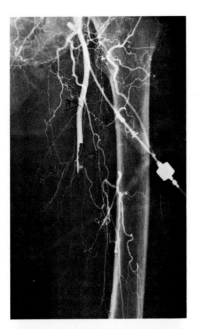

Fig. 5.10 Arterial embolism. *A 62-year-old woman with a long history of atrial fibrillation was admitted with acute ischemia of the left leg from the thigh to the foot. This film of the thigh from a femoral arteriogram demonstrates no visualization of the superficial femoral artery, a finding that could be acute or chronic in nature. The deep femoral artery (arrow 1) is occluded in the upper thigh and there is a sharply marginated, lucent filling defect just above the point of occlusion (arrow 2). This intraluminal filling defect is the key to making the diagnosis of embolus. Other suggestive findings include the abrupt cut-off of the vessel and the relative lack of collateralization distally. Given the history of atrial fibrillation, this embolus is most likely of cardiac origin.*

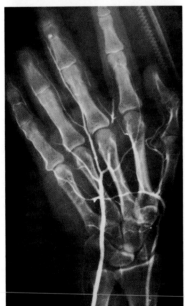

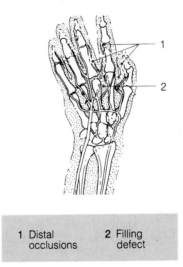

1 Distal occlusions	2 Filling defect

Fig. 5.11 Digital arterial emboli. *Small emboli frequently lodge in the most distal segments of the circulation, often manifested clinically by isolated ischemic fingers or toes. A 52-year-old woman was noted to have several blue, painful fingers a few days after subclavian artery surgery. The arteriogram demonstrates numerous distal occlusions. A filling defect can actually be seen within a metacarpal vessel, confirming the embolic nature of the problem.*

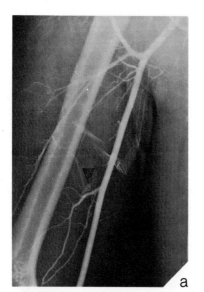

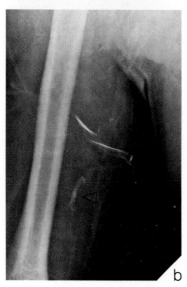

Fig. 5.12 Arterial laceration.
a This patient fell through a plate glass window and, on admission, was found to be bleeding heavily from the upper arm. The arteriogram demonstrates an irregular collection of contrast material next to one of the brachial artery branches (arrow). *b* The late-phase film demonstrates persistence of the contrast collection in the same region (arrow). These findings are typical of extravasation.

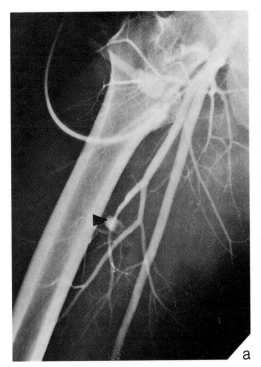

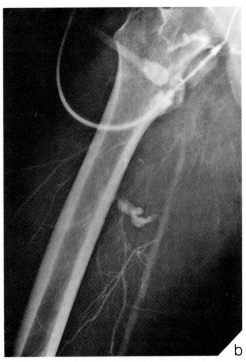

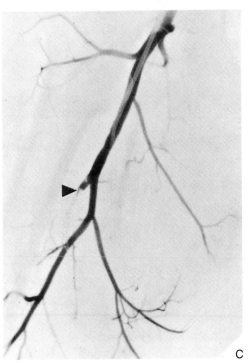

Fig. 5.13 Traumatic pseudoaneurysm.
a A patient suffered a stab wound to the inner aspect of the thigh. At that time a hematoma was noted but there was no evidence of continued bleeding. He was admitted 1 month later with an enlarging mass in the thigh following heavy exertion. The arteriogram demonstrates a pseudoaneurysm from a branch of the deep femoral artery (arrow). **b** The late-phase film shows stasis of contrast material within the pseudoaneurysm. It must be appreciated that the pseudoaneurysm is generally surrounded by a much larger hematoma than would be indicated by the opacified sac. **c** Transcatheter embolization was performed using stainless steel coils, resulting in occlusion of the traumatized branch (arrow) and control of the hemorrhage without the need for surgery.

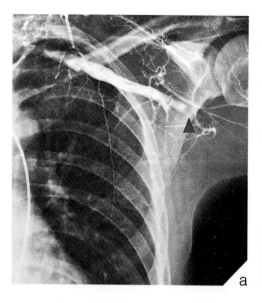

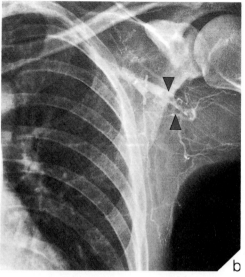

Fig. 5.14 Traumatic arterial thrombosis.
a Occasionally, vascular trauma is caused by a less obvious inciting factor. For example, this patient developed acute pain in the left upper extremity after attempting to push a heavy object. The arteriogram demonstrates abrupt occlusion of the midportion of the axillary artery (arrow). *b* The late-phase film demonstrates fresh thrombus within the vessel (arrows) *and stasis of contrast material. This type of thrombosis is presumed to be caused by extrinsic muscular trauma to the vessel. Angiographically, this would not be distinguishable from a large embolus in the axillary artery.*

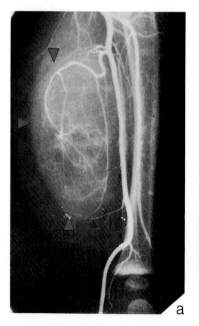

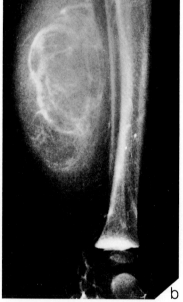

Fig. 5.15 Soft tissue sarcoma. *a* An 8-month-old child was found to have a firm mass in the calf on physical examination. The arteriogram demonstrates a hypervascular mass supplied predominantly by branches of the posterior tibial artery (arrows). *b* Dense staining is noted on the late-phase film. Surgery revealed a soft tissue sarcoma.

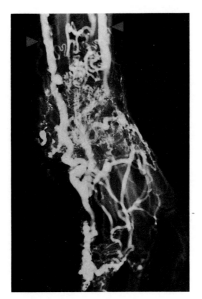

Fig. 5.16 Arteriovenous malfor-mation. *This 49-year-old man had an arteriovenous malformation of the left arm and hand since child-hood. Amputation of two fingers and a portion of the palm of the hand was performed in separate procedures. The arteriogram at this time demonstrates extensive residual malformation involving the remaining fingers, the palm, and the distal forearm. Note the marked enlargement of the radial and ulnar arteries* (arrows), *typical of vessels supplying a high-flow lesion.*

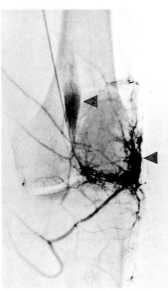

Fig. 5.17 Arteriovenous malfor-mation. *An 18-year-old man had a subtler type of arteriovenous mal-formation that caused pain in the lateral aspect of the knee. The catheter was selectively placed in one of the small geniculate branches. Numerous abnormal arteries are visible* (arrow 1) *and there is shunting into the popliteal vein* (arrow 2). *This lesion was successfully treated by emboliza-tion through the catheter and no surgery was required.*

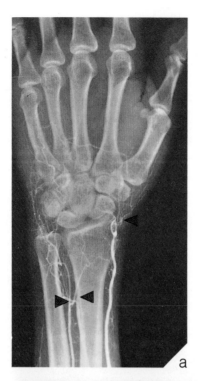

Fig. 5.18 Vasculitis. *a* This hand arteriogram of a 59-year-old man with nonspecific vasculitis demonstrates abrupt narrowing of the radial, ulnar, and interosseus arteries in the distal forearm (arrows). The vessels of the palm and digits show marked irregularity as well as segmental occlusions. ***b*** The magnification study of the fingers demonstrates these findings more dramatically (arrows). The diffuse nature of the problem and the irregularity of the vessels rule out emboli as a diagnosis, and atherosclerosis rarely involves the upper extremity in this way.

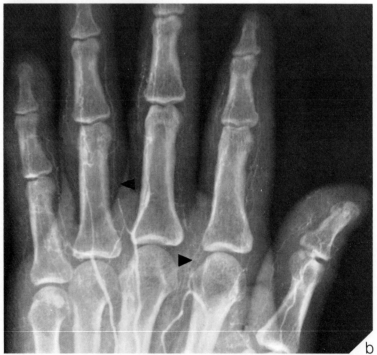

VENOGRAPHY

Despite the availability of numerous noninvasive imaging techniques, contrast venography remains the "gold standard" in the diagnosis of deep venous thrombosis (DVT). The angiographer quickly develops an appreciation of the difficulties involved in making this diagnosis clinically; certainly every swollen or painful leg does not turn out to be venous thrombosis, and the standard tests for DVT in the physical examination are notoriously unreliable. Since the diagnosis of DVT carries serious clinical implications (i.e., risk of pulmonary embolus) and involves a relatively high-risk type of treatment (anticoagulation), it is essential that the most definitive study possible be obtained.

Lower Extremity Venography

Leg venography is a simple study to perform, consisting of an injection of contrast material through an intravenous line in the foot (Figs. 5.19, 5.20). The risks are the same as for those of any study involving contrast media, with a somewhat increased danger of extravasation during the injection. Care must be taken to ensure that the intravenous line is in a good position prior to injection. With newer techniques of performing the study and the use of less concentrated contrast media, patient discomfort is minimal and the previously described complication of "post-venogram phlebitis" is uncommon. The diagnosis of DVT is seldom difficult to make with a good-quality study (Figs. 5.21–5.26).

Upper Extremity Venography

The most common indication for venography in the upper extremity is to evaluate suspected subclavian vein occlusion (Fig. 5.27). This condition can occur spontaneously after extreme muscular exertion, as a complication of central venous catheters, or as a result of extrinsic compression (e.g., by tumor). Upper extremity edema is the most common presenting symptom, and venous engorgement may also be noted.

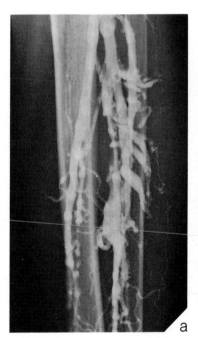
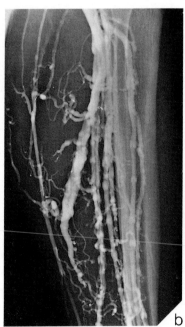
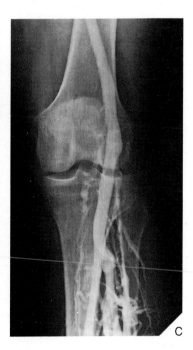

a   b   c

Fig. 5.19 Normal venous anatomy of the leg. *a, b, c* The anatomy of the venous system in the lower extremities varies much more than the corresponding arterial anatomy. This study of a normal leg demonstrates that the multiplicity of superimposed calf veins may make it difficult to exclude the presence of deep venous thrombosis (DVT). Therefore, oblique views are generally taken of this region. Interpretation is simpler at the popliteal and higher levels. Generally, the deep venous system up to at least the external iliac level can be visualized during venography.

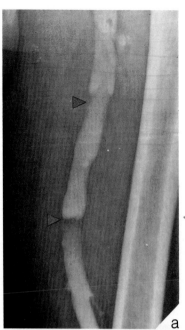

Fig. 5.20 Normal venous valves.
a, b Note the appearance of normal venous valves in the femoral vein of the thigh (*a,* arrows). *There is slight extrinsic narrowing of the iliac vein in this case due to a pelvic mass (*b,* arrows).*

a

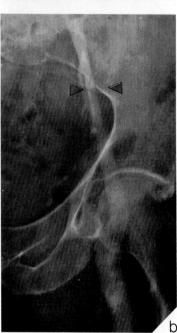

b

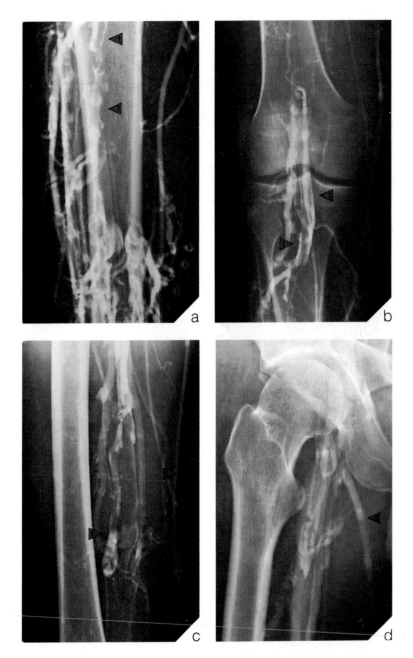

Fig. 5.21 Deep venous thrombosis (DVT). *a, b, c, d* *This venogram
sequence of the right leg demonstrates the typical findings of acute DVT
extending from the calf veins to the common femoral level. To make a
firm diagnosis, acute thrombus must be visualized within the deep veins
as seen here in the upper calf, popliteal region, and thigh (arrows 1). A
small amount of contrast generally flows around the thrombus, producing
a ghost-like appearance. Nonfilling of deep veins may suggest the diagnosis of DVT; however, this finding is not in itself sufficient to make a
diagnosis. Note the normal saphenous vein in the medial soft tissues, a
part of the superficial venous system (arrows 2).*

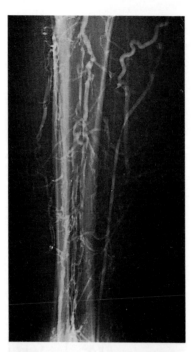

Fig. 5.22 Deep venous thrombosis. *This is another example of extensive DVT involving the calf veins. Note that almost every deep vein contains an elongated lucent filling defect representing thrombus with contrast passing around it.*

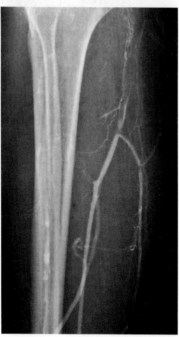

Fig. 5.23 Deep venous thrombosis. *In some cases, the deep veins may be so completely filled with thrombus that essentially all of the venous flow is diverted into the superficial veins. In this case, some clot material is also present in the superficial veins. Generally, at least one segment of the deep vessels can be seen with thrombus in the lumen. If repeated attempts show no filling of the deep system, a presumptive diagnosis of complete thrombosis can be made.*

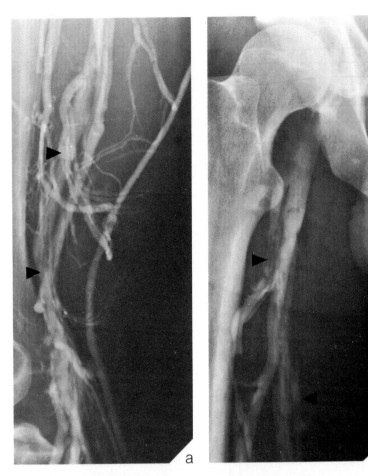

Fig. 5.24 Recanalized venous thrombus. *a, b When deep venous thrombosis is adequately treated and has clinically resolved, there usually are no abnormalities visible on follow-up venograms. Occasionally, recanalization of the thrombi will be incomplete and fibrin strands will persist in the lumen of the veins. This development produces a '"webbed" appearance consisting of fine linear defects or striations, as seen here in the veins of the popliteal and thigh region (arrows). Webbing may be associated with extensive destruction of the venous valve system and subsequent venous valvular insufficiency. Sometimes the webbing is so extensive that it is impossible to exclude completely a superimposed acute thrombosis.*

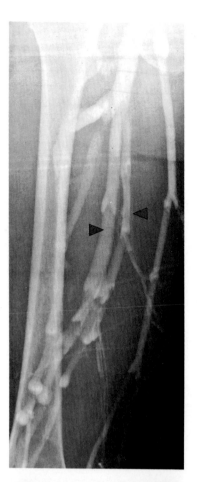

Fig. 5.25 Double femoral vein.
The anatomy of the peripheral venous system is highly variable, a fact that one must constantly bear in mind when interpreting leg venograms. In this case, there is a double femoral vein (arrows) in the thigh. While this is of no significance in itself, the diagnosis of DVT could be missed if one femoral vein thrombosed while the other remained patent.

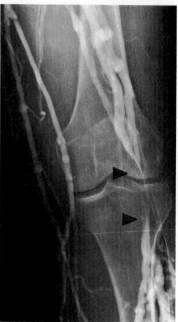

Fig. 5.26 Extrinsic compression of the popliteal vein. *Any extrinsic mass can cause displacement and compression of veins in the extremity. If the compression is severe enough, it may result in a secondary thrombosis below the site of obstruction due to stasis. In this case, there is a marked extrinsic compression of the popliteal vein (arrows). The smooth-tapered nature of the defect and the lateral displacement indicate that this is an extrinsic problem rather than intrinsic venous disease. The differential diagnosis would include soft tissue tumor, a large popliteal aneurysm, or (as in this case) a large Baker's cyst. Ultrasonography confirmed the presence of a cystic mass and a normal popliteal artery.*

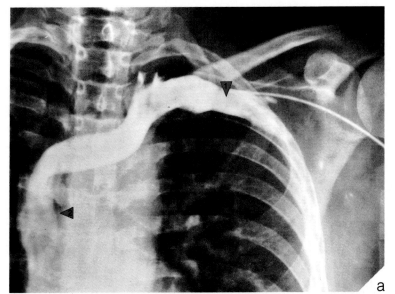

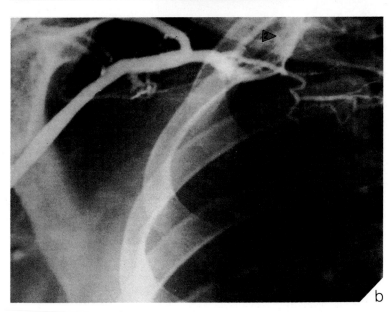

Fig. 5.27 Subclavian venography. *a* This is a normal subclavian venogram performed by inserting a catheter through an antecubital vein and passing it proximally into the distal subclavian vein. The study demonstrates a widely patent subclavian vein (arrow 1) draining into the superior vena cava (arrow 2). ***b*** This film demonstrates the typical findings in subclavian vein thrombosis with complete occlusion of the subclavian vein and filling of collateral venous pathways (arrow 2). The collaterals typically drain through the jugular circulation and less commonly through the chest wall.

CHAPTER SIX

Lymphangiography

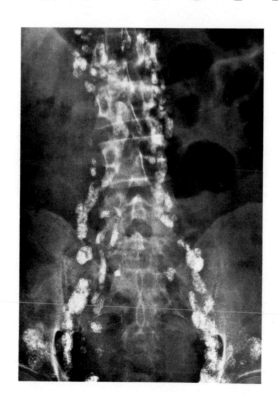

Lymphangiography, a rather involved procedure for visualizing the lymph nodes in the abdomen and pelvis, is usually employed in the diagnostic work-up of malignant disease, especially pelvic tumors and lymphomas. With the advent of CT and ultrasound, which can demonstrate the presence or absence of gross lymph node enlargement, lymphangiography is performed much less often. However, when the CT scan is equivocal or normal, a lymphangiogram may be helpful in

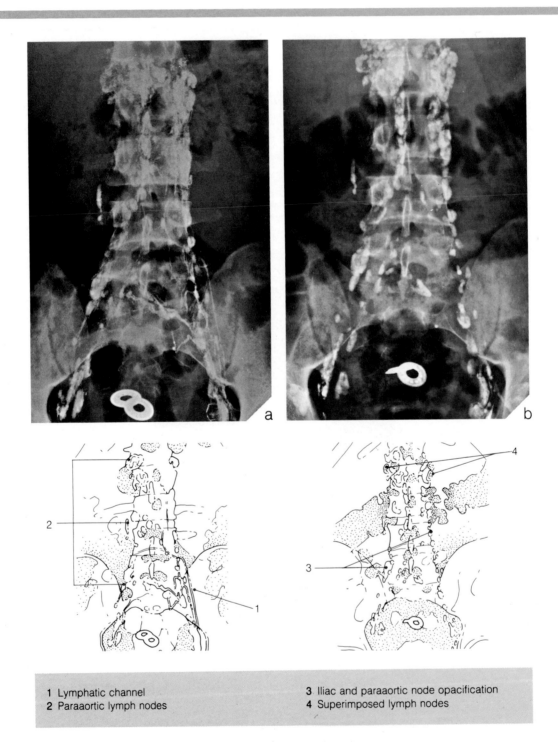

1 Lymphatic channel	3 Iliac and paraaortic node opacification
2 Paraaortic lymph nodes	4 Superimposed lymph nodes

showing subtle abnormalities, such as filling defects or changes in texture, that could indicate the presence of malignant disease.

The study involves a minor surgical procedure, to permit direct exposure and cannulation of the lymphatic channels on the dorsum of each foot and slow injection of an oily iodinated contrast medium. Films of the abdomen and pelvis are obtained immediately after completion of the injection in what is called the channel phase; another set of films is taken 24 hours later, in the nodal phase, when contrast has left the lymphatic channels and lodged in the pelvic and paraaortic nodes. The contrast remains in these nodes for several months and can be seen on plain radiographs.

Normal lymph nodes vary markedly in appearance but tend to have an elongated bean shape and a dense granular texture (Fig. 6.1). They are intimately associated with the iliac arteries, and longitudinal grooves, representing vascular impressions, may normally be seen in the pelvic nodes.

Malignant involvement of the lymph nodes may result in nodal enlargement, changes in the internal texture (e.g., the "foamy" nodes seen in lymphoma; Fig. 6.2), sharply marginated filling defects (usually associated with metastatic disease; Fig. 6.3), or complete replacement of the node by tumor. The latter may result in a complete lack of opacification, but the diagnosis can sometimes be suggested by obstruction of lymph channels with persistent filling of dilated channels on the nodal-phase films, which are normally free of contrast by that time.

Lymphangiography is also performed occasionally to investigate suspected nonmalignant lymphatic problems, such as congenital abnormalities, unexplained edema, or involvement of the lymphatic system by trauma (Fig. 6.4).

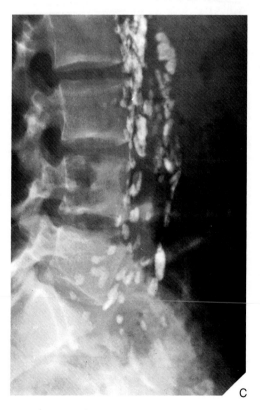

C

Fig. 6.1 Normal lymphangiogram. *In a study performed as part of the diagnostic evaluation of a 19-year-old man with known Hodgkin's disease in the mediastinum, these normal lymphangiograms were obtained.* **a** *A channel-phase film obtained immediately following contrast injection through the lymphatics in both feet clearly demonstrates the lymphatic channels, as well as early filling of the iliac and paraaortic lymph nodes. Little diagnostic information is usually available in channel-phase films except for the suggestion of obstructed or displaced channels.* **b** *On a nodal-phase film, obtained 24 hours after injection, there is good opacification of the iliac and paraaortic nodes. Note the normal elongated bean shape of the lymph nodes with their homogenous yet somewhat granular consistency. When many lymph nodes are superimposed on each other, one can appreciate the difficulty in ruling out a filling defect.* **c** *Lateral, as shown here, and oblique films can usually separate the nodes enough to determine the presence of defects.*

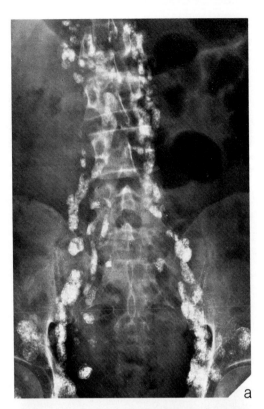

a

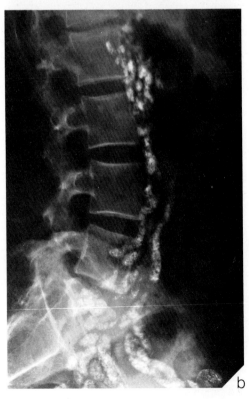

b

Fig. 6.2 Hodgkin's disease. *a, b Positive nodal-phase lymphangiogram of a 35-year-old man with known Hodgkin's disease demonstrates enlargement of all of the iliac and paraaortic nodes. More important is the alteration in the normal texture of the nodes, with numerous small filling defects and a generalized "foamy" appearance. These findings are typical of lymphomatous involvement, confirmed in this case at laparotomy.*

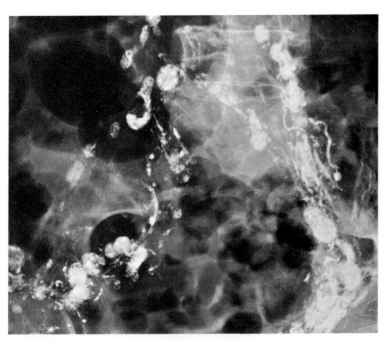

Fig. 6.3 Metastatic carcinoma.
*Positive lymphangiogram in a
patient with metastatic cervical
carcinoma demonstrates a sharply
marginated filling defect (arrow)
suggestive of metastatic disease.
There is considerable variation in
the lymphangiographic appearance of lymphoma and metastatic
disease; the two are not always
distinguishable.*

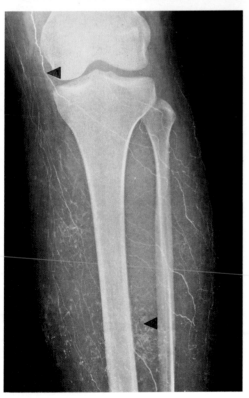

Fig. 6.4 Lymphatic obstruction. *In a 20-year-old woman
being evaluated for unexplained edema of the left leg,
venograms (not shown) were negative. This channel phase
lymphangiogram demonstrates the fine caliber of normal
lymphatic vessels in the extremities (arrow 1). The irregular
collections of contrast material scattered through the soft tissues (arrow 2) are consistent with dermal backflow generally
encountered in lymphatic obstruction. In this case, severe
inflammatory disease caused obstructive changes in the
pelvic nodes on this side.*

SECTION II:

Interventional Radiology

Interventional radiology has emerged as an exciting and rapidly expanding subspecialty of diagnostic radiology. It presents the unique challenges and frustrations inherent in the care of critically ill patients while offering the rewards of successful and often dramatic intervention in the course of an illness. This subspecialty has evolved from the utilization of angiographic catheters for the delivery of therapeutic agents within the vascular system to include the use of cross-sectional imaging for organ biopsy and abscess drainage. Angiographic techniques have been adopted for intervention in the gut, hepatobiliary, and urinary systems. New techniques emerge at a rapid pace, challenging the interventional radiologist to keep pace with the growth of the subspecialty.

The diagnostic radiologist is now a central figure in the therapy of critically ill patients. With this new role comes the responsibility to provide these procedures at times which have been previously considered "off hours" for radiologists. The interventional radiologist must be cognizant of all therapeutic options in order to advise the clinician when radiologic intervention is appropriate. Since many of these procedures are new, the radiologist has the responsibility to evaluate their risks and benefits in a scientific manner before incorporating them into his current therapeutic armamentarium.

CHAPTER SEVEN

Percutaneous Fine Needle Aspiration Biopsy

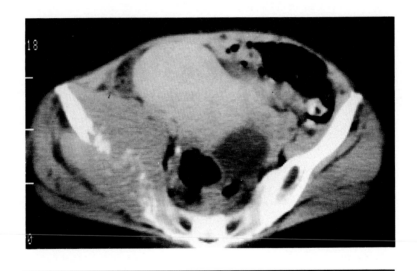

Percutaneous fine needle aspiration biopsy (FNAB) is a rapid, safe, and effective method for obtaining tissue for diagnosis of masses located in virtually any part of the body. The procedure eliminates the need for surgical procedures that would be performed only for tumor diagnosis. Cross-sectional imaging techniques (CT and ultrasound) precisely localize masses in solid organs, in the retroperitoneum, and in the mediastinum; they also provide precise needle guidance for the biopsy procedure. Biopsy needles constructed with thin walls and cutting edges ensure that tissue cores can be obtained from needles as fine as 21 gauge.

INDICATIONS

FNAB is indicated in a variety of clinical settings. It can be used to document metastatic disease in patients with a known primary and to exclude the possibility of a second primary. It can also be used to establish a precise tissue diagnosis, which facilitates the choice of appropriate therapy. In the lung, for example, a diagnosis of lymphoma or small-cell carcinoma by FNAB may lead to non-surgical therapy (Fig. 7.1).

While FNAB is often used to differentiate benign from malignant disease, it must be remembered that the diagnosis of malignancy is not made in 3 to 14 percent of the patients with malignant disease. In patients with obvious metastatic disease in whom the primary tumor is not apparent, FNAB can direct and tailor the diagnostic work-up or provide tissue before therapy is begun. In patients with a known malignancy who are being reevaluated during therapy, FNAB frequently eliminates the need for surgical restaging procedures.

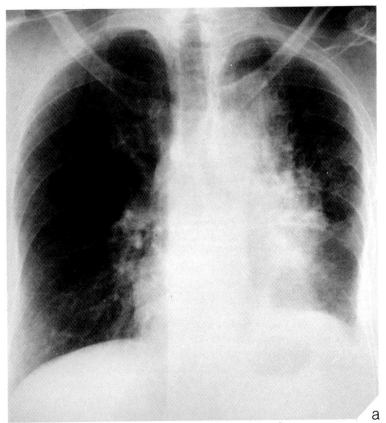

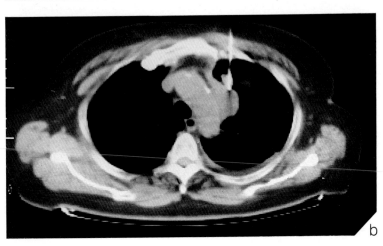

Fig. 7.1 CT-guided biopsy of a mediastinal mass. *a Chest radiograph demonstrates a mass involving the left hilar region with left upper lobe collapse. **b** A CT scan shows left paraaortic mediastinal adenopathy. Since this region cannot be sampled by routine mediastinoscopy, a CT-directed mediastinal biopsy was performed (arrow indicates biopsy needle entering the mass). The biopsy revealed small cell carcinoma and the patient was treated with chemotherapy.*

TECHNIQUE

FNAB is performed with the patient receiving local anesthesia and, occasionally, mild sedation. The procedure is usually done with a 21-gauge cutting needle, although needles as small as 23 gauge or as large as 18 or 19 gauge may be used. Lung and bone lesions, as well as lymph nodes opacified by lymphangiography, are generally biopsied under direct fluoroscopic guidance (Figs. 7.2, 7.3); biplane fluoroscopy aids in biopsy of very small lung lesions. CT or ultrasound is utilized for most other biopsies. Ultrasound has the advantage of providing continuous monitoring of the needle tip and is particularly useful for biopsies of the liver, kidney, and pelvic organs (Fig. 7.4). CT is usually necessary for pancreatic, retroperitoneal, and mediastinal biopsies (Figs. 7.5, 7.6). Although the bowel is routinely traversed by the needle during abdominal biopsies, complications rarely arise when 21-gauge or smaller needles are used.

Although needle selection frequently reflects the prejudices of the physician, certain principles seem fundamental. The larger the caliber of the biopsy needle, the greater the complication rate; this becomes a significant problem when 18-gauge or larger needles are used. Beveled small-bore needles have a better yield than nonbeveled small-bore needles of similar design. Certain designs (e.g., Franseen trephine, slotted, and cutting-edge needles) provide better specimens than spinal or Chiba-type needles (Fig. 7.7).

Once the biopsy needle is in contact with the tumor mass, suction is applied to the hub of the needle with a 10- or 20-mL syringe. With full suction applied, the needle is gently agitated vertically over a distance of 1 to 2 cm. Alternatively, the needle can be rotated in the lesion while the tip is advanced over a short distance to provide a cutting action. Immediate preparation of slides, as well as proper handling of the specimen for cell-block preparation and special staining, are essential to the success of FNAB. It is therefore extremely important that a cytotechnologist be present during the procedure. Because special stains may be needed to distinguish between various neoplasms, close cooperation between radiologist and cytopathologist is also essential.

Whereas the biopsy needles used in the past for FNAB provided hypocellular specimens that required sophisticated cytologic diagnosis, modern biopsy needles generally yield enough tissue for cell blocks and histologic diagnosis. With disorders requiring architectural analysis for diagnosis (e.g., cirrhosis), however, the specimens needed are larger than FNAB can provide.

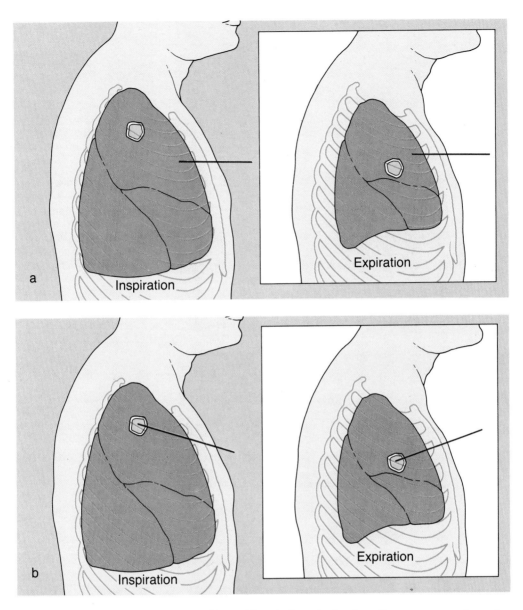

Fig. 7.2 Method of determining needle position during single-plane fluoroscopy. *a A needle that is superimposed on a pulmonary nodule but is not at the required depth moves independently of the nodule. b When the needle is in the nodule, needle and nodule move as one.*

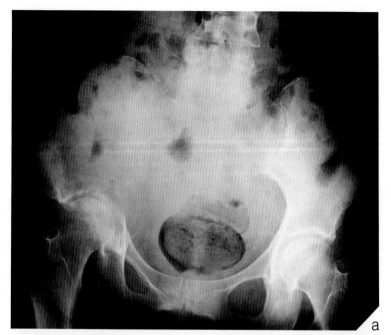

Fig. 7.3 Diagnosis of bone lymphoma by FNAB. *a Plain film of the pelvis reveals a poorly circumscribed lytic lesion involving the right ilium of this 43-year-old woman. b CT of the pelvis demonstrates destruction of the ilium with a large soft-tissue component. In addition, there is an enlarged uterus. Since it seemed unlikely that the bone destruction was due to metastases from a primary uterine malignancy, FNAB of the bone lesion was performed under fluoroscopic guidance. Lymphoma was diagnosed from the aspirate, and the patient was treated with radiation therapy. The uterine enlargement was secondary to fibroids.*

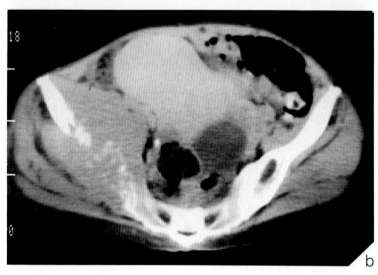

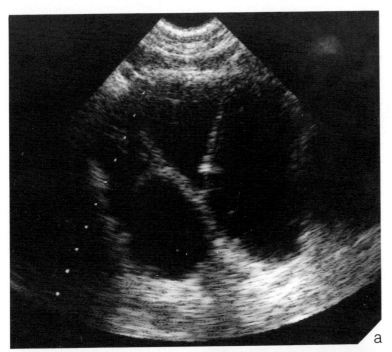

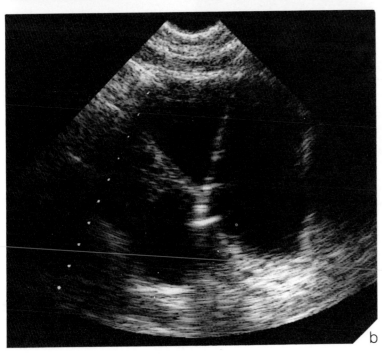

Fig. 7.4 Ultrasonically guided biopsy of an ovarian mass.
*Pelvic ultrasound demonstrates a cystic left ovarian mass in this 64-year-old woman. A transvesical approach for aspiration biopsy allows accurate needle monitoring as the ovary is approached (**a**) and as the cystic lesion is penetrated (**b**). The diagnosis from the aspirate was adenocarcinoma of the ovary.*

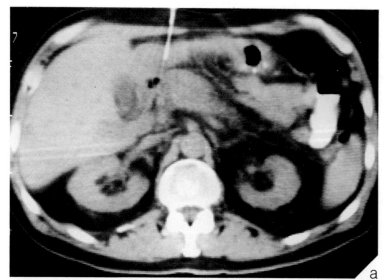

Fig. 7.5 CT-guided biopsy of pancreatic mass. *The precise guidance provided by CT is demonstrated on these sequential images of a percutaneous biopsy of a mass in the head of the pancreas.* **a** *The initial direction of the biopsy needle will miss the 2-cm mass by 1 cm.* **b** *After the needle is redirected, the mass is successfully aspirated.*

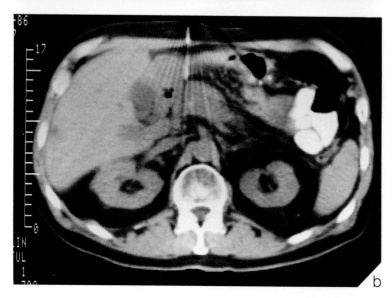

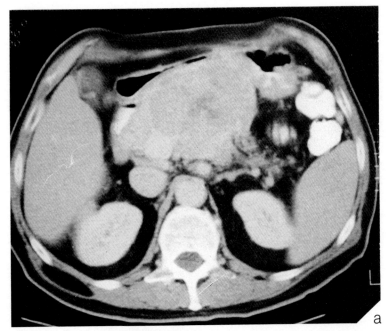

a

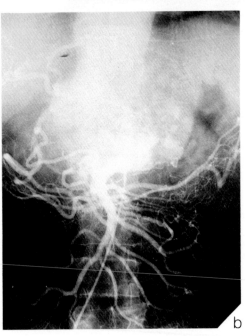

b

Fig. 7.6 Percutaneous biopsy of a pancreatic tumor. *This otherwise asymptomatic patient presented with an abdominal mass. **a** CT demonstrates a very large, well-marginated mass in the head and body of the pancreas. **b** A superior mesenteric artery angiogram shows that the mass is hypervascular. Since it was unlikely that this represented adenocarcinoma of the exocrine pancreas, FNAB was performed, confirming the clinical and radiologic diagnosis of a nonfunctioning islet-cell carcinoma.*

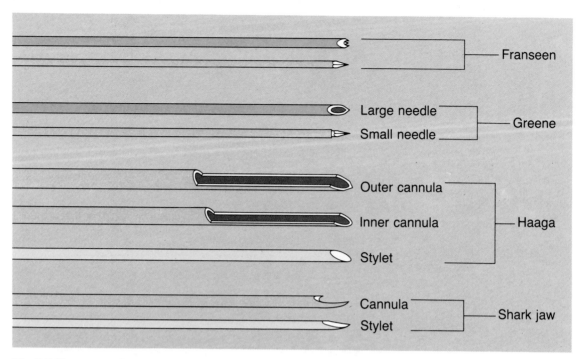

Fig. 7.7 Biopsy needles. *Shown are a few of the many available aspiration biopsy needles.*

RESULTS

Although masses in most organs can be successfully biopsied by means of fine-needle techniques, there are organ-specific differences in the diagnostic yield. In several reported series, the sensitivity of FNAB in the diagnosis of lung malignancy is 85 to 95 percent. The sensitivity and specificity are less for benign lesions. Fine-needle aspiration often yields a nonspecific tissue diagnosis (e.g., "fibrosis" or "inflammation") in such cases; without a specific diagnosis, such as granuloma or hamartoma, malignancy cannot be excluded.

For lesions of the liver, kidney, and pancreas, the diagnostic yield of FNAB ranges from 70 percent to higher than 90 percent. The sensitivity for pancreatic carcinoma is closer to the low end of this range, which reflects the sampling error induced by the inflammatory changes that often accompany pancreatic malignancies and the hypocellularity of the specimens obtained from this scirrhous neoplasm.

In patients with metastatic epithelial malignancies, percutaneous lymph-node biopsy yields results similar to those of percutaneous abdominal biopsies in general. FNAB is less satisfactory in the diagnosis of primary lymph-node neoplasms: the sensitivity ranges from 50 to 75 percent in patients with well-differentiated lymphosarcoma and Hodgkin's disease (Fig. 7.8). Patients with suspected Hodgkin's disease or lymphoma are more appropriately diagnosed by incisional biopsy, particularly when palpable nodes are present. FNAB is, however, of considerable value in the restaging of patients in whom a diagnosis of Hodgkin's disease or lymphoma has been confirmed.

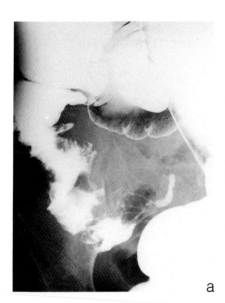

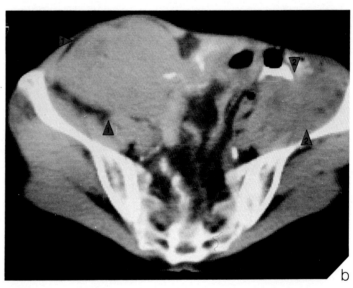

a

b

Fig. 7.8 Diagnosis of abdominal lymphoma by FNAB. *a Spot film from a barium enema demonstrates a large right lower quadrant mass infiltrating the cecum. b A CT scan of the abdomen reveals a large mass involving the colon* (arrows 1). *Abnormal lymph nodes* (arrows 2) *are seen in the left iliac region. These findings prompted FNAB, which revealed poorly differentiated lymphoma. The patient was treated medically.*

COMPLICATIONS

Serious complications of FNAB are infrequent. For this reason, I routinely perform percutaneous biopsies on an outpatient basis, observing the patient in the radiology department for several hours after completion of the procedure.

Lung and mediastinal biopsies are complicated by pneumothorax in as many as 25 percent of patients; however, a chest tube is required in fewer than 10 percent. I have employed a modification of the technique that further decreases the incidence of pneumothorax (Fig. 7.9). Hemoptysis occurs in fewer than 10 percent of patients.

Bleeding is a potential complication of any per-

cutaneous abdominal biopsy. It usually is clinically silent, and it seldom requires intervention. Although the bowel is routinely traversed in the course of abdominal biopsies, peritonitis due to leakage of bowel contents is rare. Caution must, however, be exercised in traversing bowel that is compromised by tumor, for leakage of bowel contents is more likely in this setting.

Tumor seeding has been reported as a complication of FNAB, but it is a distinctly unusual one. There is no convincing evidence that FNAB decreases survival in patients with malignant neoplasms.

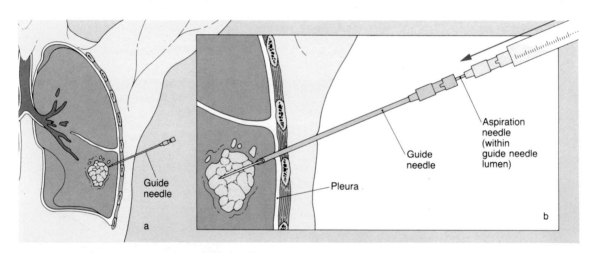

Fig. 7.9 Coaxial method of lung biopsy. *a The visceral pleura is punctured by a guide needle, which is then advanced into the lung and positioned just above the near surface of the lung mass. **b** A smaller aspiration needle is passed into the lumen of the* *guide needle and advanced into the tumor. Since multiple biopsies can be obtained after a single pass of the guide needle, multiple punctures of the pleura are unnecessary.*

CHAPTER EIGHT

Percutaneous Drainage of Intraabdominal Abscesses

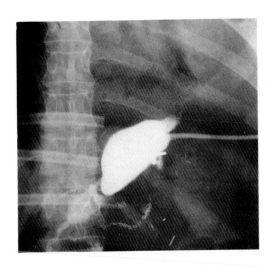

The ability to drain intraabdominal abscesses successfully through percutaneous techniques, thereby eliminating the need for surgical drainage in critically ill patients, has been heralded as one of the major medical advances of the past decade. Initially restricted to abscesses immediately adjacent to the abdominal wall, percutaneous abscess drainage (PAD) is now a realistic option for almost all intraabdominal abscesses, including visceral and interloop abscesses.

PAD relies on the precise anatomic detail achievable by modern cross-sectional imaging techniques, CT in particular. Besides being a sensitive method for detecting abdominal abscesses, CT is capable of individually distinguishing multiple abscesses, all of which must be drained if the procedure is to succeed. By accurately depicting the normal anatomy in the vicinity of the abscess, CT allows the interventional radiologist to plan a drainage route that avoids bowel and solid viscera. The choice of drainage route varies with the location of the abscess. Transperitoneal and extraperitoneal routes are the most commonly used; a transvaginal or transrectal approach may be necessary for drainage of a hard-to-reach pelvic abscess. In general, the drainage catheter should not traverse bowel or abdominal viscera; however, the transgastric route has been successfully employed for drainage of pancreatic pseudocysts, and successful transhepatic drainage of subhepatic abscesses has been reported.

If PAD is to be safe and successful, meticulous patient selection and aftercare are crucial. It is therefore essential that the interventional radiologist and the surgeon collaborate closely, both before and after the procedure.

TECHNIQUE AND AFTERCARE

Although the planning of the drainage procedure usually depends on a preliminary CT scan, the actual placement of the needle can be done under the guidance either of CT or of real-time ultrasound. The latter technique allows continual monitoring of needle position. Ultrasound is best suited to drainage of superficial abscesses, abscesses in solid viscera, and abscesses not surrounded by bowel. In patients with these conditions, it can significantly decrease procedure time.

With the patient under local anesthesia and mildly sedated, a 20-gauge needle is carefully directed into the intraabdominal fluid in such a way as to avoid adjacent bowel and solid viscera

(Fig. 8.1). Once the fluid collection has been entered, a sample of fluid is aspirated so that its nature can be determined. (Not every fluid collection is an abscess: benign serous collections are seen one week after abdominal surgery in as many as 20 percent of patients.)

If diagnostic aspiration indicates the presence of an abscess, a drainage catheter is placed into the abscess cavity. In the widely used Seldinger technique (Fig. 8.2), a 0.18-in. guidewire is passed through the 20-gauge diagnostic needle. Progressively larger dilating catheters and guidewires are then introduced, enlarging the drainage tract until an 8- to 16-French drainage catheter can be advanced into the abscess cavity. Once the drainage catheter is in place, the abscess is completely evacuated of pus and irrigated with a mixture of saline and Betadine (Fig. 8.3). Drainage of complex and multi-loculated abscesses frequently requires several catheters (Fig. 8.4).

A one-step trocar technique is often used as an alternative to the Seldinger method. In this technique, a trocar catheter system consisting of a cannula, a pointed stylet, and a pigtail catheter is introduced alongside the diagnostic needle (Fig. 8.5). Tandem insertion ensures that the tip of the stylet is positioned at exactly the same depth and location as the tip of the diagnostic needle, which in turn ensures that the drainage catheter is correctly placed when the stylet is withdrawn. The one-step trocar method also eliminates the need for tract dilatation and guidewire manipulation within the abscess cavity, thereby reducing the likelihood of septicemia and cavity perforation. It can be used for some collections for which the Seldinger technique is unsuited, such as cul-de-sac abscesses (Figs. 8.6, 8.7).

Antibiotic coverage is initiated at the time of abscess drainage and generally is continued as long as the drainage catheter remains in place (one to two weeks for most "routine" abscesses). Abscesses that communicate with the bowel necessitate much longer periods of catheter drainage: in such cases, the catheter must remain in place until the fistula closes, which may take several months (Fig. 8.8).

Successful abscess drainage is heralded by prompt defervescence and return of the patient's white blood cell (WBC) count to normal. The fluid draining from the catheter rapidly changes from grossly purulent to serous or serosanguinous. Once the patient's body temperature and WBC count have returned to normal (usually one to three days after drainage), he or she may be managed as an outpatient with the drainage catheter in place.

If there is an adequate clinical response to catheter drainage, frequent imaging with ultrasound or CT is unnecessary. Contrast studies of the abscess cavity are not routinely performed, and in general are done only if there are grounds for suspecting a bowel fistula (for instance, if the daily drainage volume is greater than 50 to 100 mL).

Persistent fever may indicate the presence of a loculated collection that is not being adequately drained. Contrast injection of a multiloculated or complex abscess cavity, followed by CT scanning, will determine whether loculated spaces communicate with each other and how many additional drainage catheters are needed.

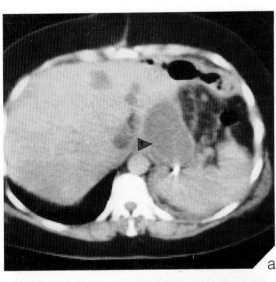

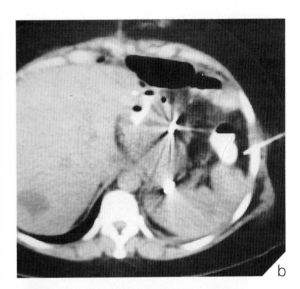

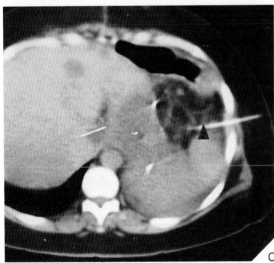

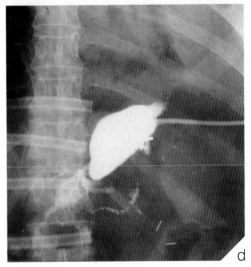

Fig. 8.1 Transperitoneal drainage of upper abdominal interloop abscess. *An upper abdominal abscess developed in this patient after a gastric resection.*
a–c A CT scan demonstrates an upper abdominal abscess (arrow 1). The gastric remnant, liver, spleen, colon, and small bowel loops surround the abscess. The tip of the diagnostic needle (arrow 2) can be seen. *Under CT guidance (**b,c**), it was necessary to redirect the diagnostic needle several times so that it could puncture the abscess without traversing bowel or surrounding viscera. **d** A contrast study after partial drainage of the abscess shows no communication with the bowel.*

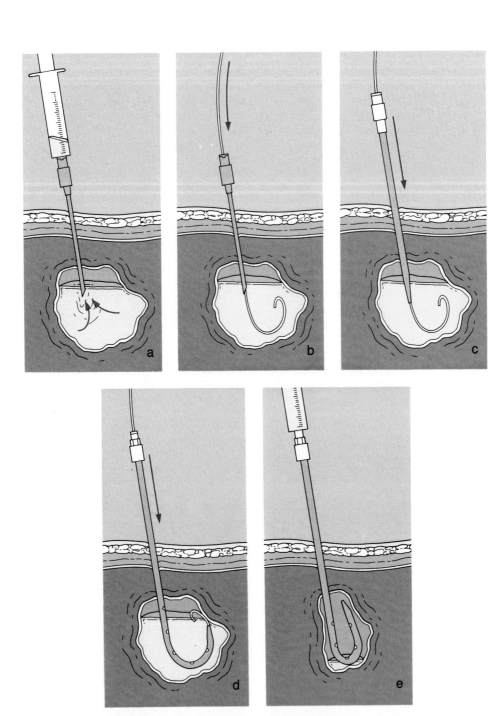

Fig. 8.2 Seldinger method of catheter placement. *a* *A 20-gauge or larger needle is advanced percutaneously into the abscess cavity. **b** After satisfactory placement of the needle is confirmed by aspiration of the abscess contents, a .018- to .035-in. guidewire is advanced into the abscess cavity. **c** A stiff catheter is passed over the guidewire to dilate the drainage tract. Progressively larger dilators are then introduced over the guidewire until the tract is large enough to accept the drainage catheter. **d** An 8- to 12-French drainage catheter with multiple side holes is passed over the guidewire into the abscess cavity. **e** The guidewire is withdrawn, and the catheter is left in the abscess cavity.*

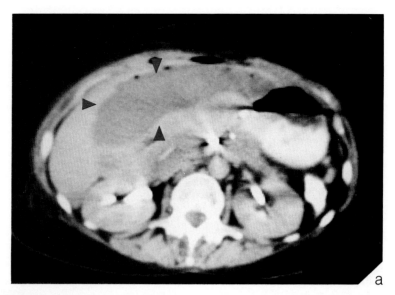

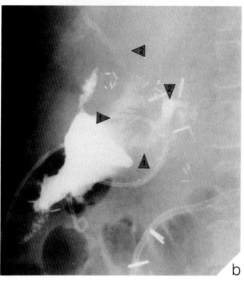

Fig. 8.3 Transperitoneal drainage of a subhepatic abscess. *This patient developed a right upper quadrant abscess after a Whipple procedure.* **a** *A CT scan shows a large subhepatic abscess (arrows).* **b** *A contrast injection after successful PAD reveals a small residual abscess cavity communicating with the duodenum (arrows 1) and the biliary tree (arrows 2), which confirms leakage from the pancreaticoduodenal anastomosis. Catheter drainage was continued for two additional months to allow time for the fistula to close.*

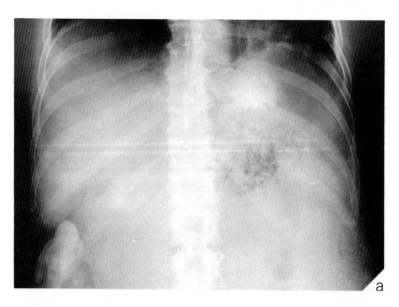

a

Fig. 8.4 Transperitoneal drainage of pancreatic abscess. *a A plain film shows a bubbly gas pattern in the left upper quadrant that represents gas within a pancreatic abscess. b CT scan of the upper abdomen shows multiple loculated collections of gas and fluid resulting from partial diges- tion of tissue by pancreatic enzymes and secondary infection. Note the retroperitoneal and perinephric fluid collections secondary to the inflam- matory process. c Repeat CT shows two 12-French drainage catheters in the area of the infected pancreas. Although two days had elapsed since the placement of the drainage catheters, very little of this complex abscess had drained, and the patient's condition had not improved. This case illustrates the difficulty of draining pancreatic abscesses completely.*

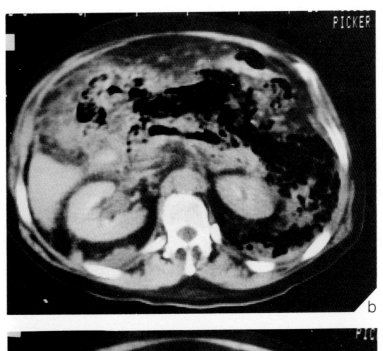

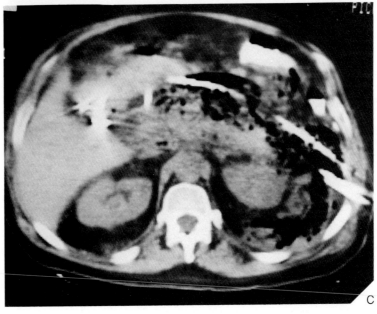

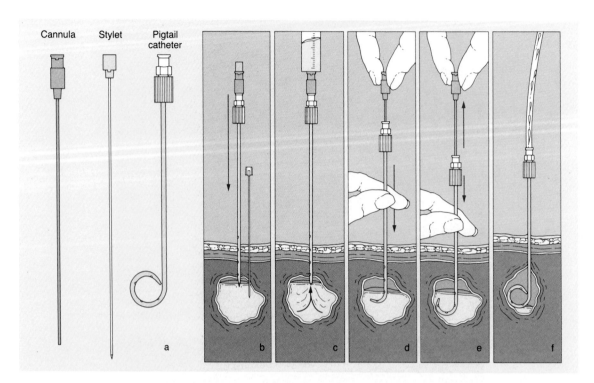

Fig. 8.5 One-step trocar catheter placement. *a The trocar system includes an 18-gauge or larger cannula with a pointed stylet which is loaded into a multiholed pigtail catheter. b After the tip of the 20-gauge diagnostic needle has been positioned within the abscess cavity, the trocar system is introduced alongside the diagnostic needle through a small skin incision. Under CT or sonographic guidance, the trocar system is thrust in one pass into the most superficial aspect of the abscess cavity, exactly duplicating the course and depth of the diagnostic needle. c The stylet is removed, and a few milliliters of the abscess contents is aspirated to confirm that the tip of the cannula is within the abscess cavity. d The drainage catheter is advanced over the cannula into the abscess cavity, e the cannula is withdrawn, and f the catheter is attached to a gravity drainage system.*

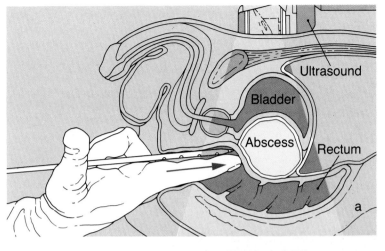

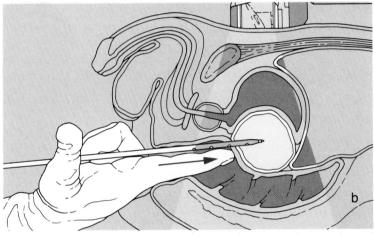

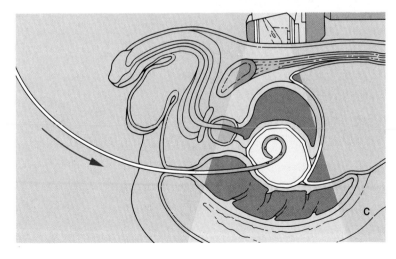

Fig. 8.6 Transrectal drainage of pelvic abscess (one-step trocar method). *Cul-de-sac abscesses are frequently surrounded by bowel and bladder, in which case transperitoneal drainage is not feasible. Transrectal drainage, using continuous real-time ultra-sound monitoring, may eliminate the need for laparotomy in these difficult cases. **a** With the trocar system positioned on the ventral surface of the index finger, the operator introduces both into the rectum and advances the finger until the lower margin of the cul-de-sac abscess can be palpated. **b** Under continuous ultrasonic guidance, the trocar system is thrust into the central portion of the abscess cavity. **c** Holding the stylet in place, the operator advances the catheter into the abscess cavity until the drainage catheter assumes its pigtailed con-figuration, which indicates that it is in satisfactory position. (Adapted with permission from Nosher et al: AJR 146:1047, 1986.).*

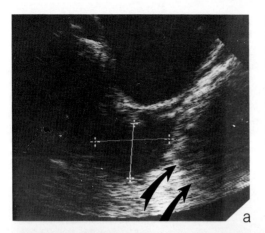

Fig. 8.7 Transrectal abscess drainage.
Longitudinal sonograms. **a** *Lines indicate the cul-de-sac abscess. The operator's finger appears as an echogenic focus* (arrows). **b** *The tip of the trocar is indicated by echoes* (arrow) *in the abscess cavity.* **c** *After partial drainage, the abscess is much smaller. The drainage catheter* (arrow) *remains in the abscess cavity. (Reproduced with permission from Nosher et al: AJR 146:1047, 1986.)*

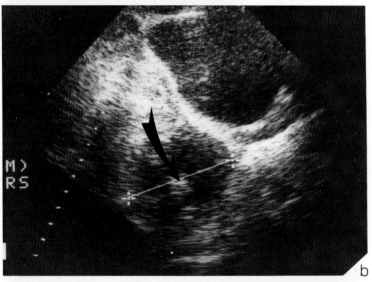

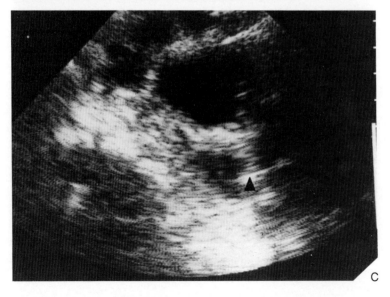

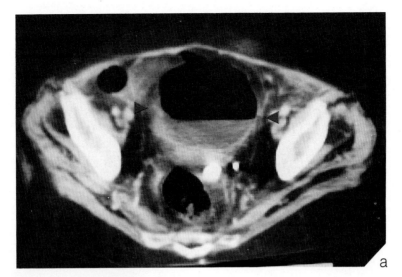

a

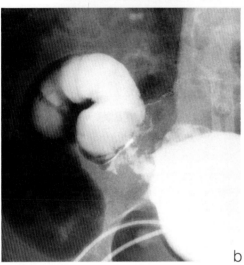

b

Fig. 8.8 Pelvic abscess with bowel fistula.
*After this patient underwent an ileocolostomy,
a pelvic abscess developed.* ***a*** *A CT scan of
the pelvis shows a large midline pelvic abscess
(arrows) with an air/fluid level. After successful
initial drainage of the cavity, large volumes of
nonpurulent fluid continued to drain from it,
suggesting the presence of a bowel fistula.*
b *A contrast study shows a fistula between
the abscess and the ileum. An additional three
weeks of catheter drainage were needed
before the fistula closed.*

COMPLICATIONS

Complications occur in fewer than 10 percent of cases and are usually minor. Serious and potentially fatal complications of PAD include organ failure due to incompletely treated sepsis, bouts of sepsis related to catheter placement or manipulation, early or late bleeding, inadvertent puncture of adjacent bowel or viscera, and inadvertent catheter expulsion.

RESULTS

The success of PAD depends on the nature of the abscess, where it is located, and whether multiple abscess cavities are present. PAD is successful in more than 90 percent of patients with unilocular abscesses containing nonviscous fluid that is free of substantial debris. The success rate decreases with the complexity of the abscess: multiloculated abscesses, abscesses that communicate with bowel, and intrasplenic or pancreatic abscesses account for most treatment failures. The failure rate for drainage of pancreatic abscesses, the least

successful drainage procedure, is higher than 50 percent. (This procedure should be differentiated from drainage of infected pancreatic pseudocysts, which carries a much higher success rate.)

Although the results of PAD and those of conventional surgical drainage are comparable, PAD has several important advantages. First, it obviates general anesthesia and surgery in critically ill patients. Second, it eliminates the morbidity and prolonged recovery period associated with any laparotomy, thereby decreasing the length of the hospital stay and reducing the utilization of hospital resources.

OTHER APPLICATIONS OF PERCUTANEOUS DRAINAGE

The same techniques used for PAD can be used to drain lymphocysts, pancreatic pseudocysts (Fig. 8.9), bilomas, cystic metastases, and other intraabdominal fluid collections. Complications of these procedures include secondary infection of sterile cavities and hemorrhage.

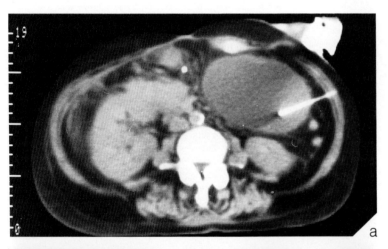

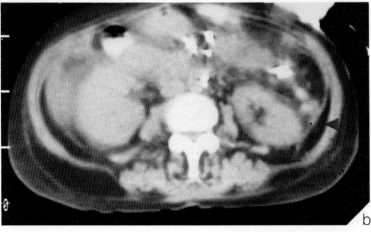

Fig. 8.9 Transperitoneal drainage of pancreatic pseudocyst. a *A CT scan shows that the tip of the 20-gauge needle is in the pseudocyst.* **b** *A repeat CT scan after complete evacuation of the pseudocyst by the one-step trocar technique shows the 8-French drainage catheter (arrows) in place.*

*P*ercutaneous Transluminal Angioplasty

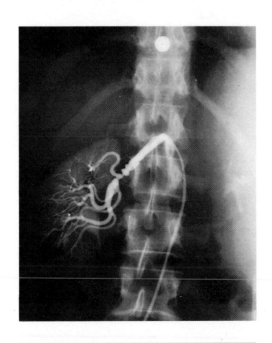

Percutaneous transluminal angioplasty (PTA) is a procedure in which a controlled vascular injury is used to dilate a stenotic or occluded blood vessel. In carefully selected patients, PTA can correct these lesions as effectively as surgical bypass or endarterectomy. The procedure grew out of the pioneering efforts of Charles Dotter, who dilated arterial lesions by passing progressively larger catheters through the area of stenosis. With the introduction of the balloon dilatation catheter (Fig. 9.1) by Andreas Grüntzig, PTA became a safe, technically easy, and effective alternative to surgery. Although virtually every major artery in the body, as well as the superior and inferior venae cavae and vascular grafts, has been dilated, success rates vary, depending on patient selection and the location of the vessel being dilated.

TECHNIQUE

After a preliminary diagnostic arteriogram or successful puncture of the access artery, the patient undergoes anticoagulation therapy with 5000 to 6000 U of heparin administered intraarterially. Under fluoroscopic guidance, a straight angiographic guidance or a J-shaped guidewire with a floppy end is passed through the area of stenosis or occlusion. This must be done with considerable care to ensure intraluminal passage of the guidewire. When the stenosis is eccentric, a curved catheter can be used to direct the guidewire through the vessel lumen. If the vessel is occluded, the tip of the diagnostic catheter should be positioned in the distal portion of the narrowed segment; an injection of contrast material will delineate the course of the vessel lumen, thus facilitating passage of the guidewire.

Once the guidewire has been successfully passed, a diagnostic catheter of the same outside diameter as the balloon dilatation catheter is advanced beyond the narrowed segment to provide initial dilatation of the area. The diagnostic catheter is then removed, and a balloon dilatation catheter is passed into the narrowed segment. The diameter of the inflated balloon should match that of the uninvolved artery immediately distal to the lesion (Fig. 9.2). Because no provision is made for magnification on the diagnostic arteriogram, the balloon is purposely oversized by about 10 percent, so that the arterial lumen is slightly overdistended when the balloon is fully inflated.

The length of the balloon is determined by the length of the lesion; if possible, the balloon should be slightly longer than the lesion to be dilated. Opaque markers at both ends of the balloon ensure accurate placement at the site of vascular abnormality. The balloon is inflated to a pressure of 4 to 5 atm, which is maintained for 20 to 30 seconds; repeated inflations are frequently necessary. There is a "waist" in the inflated balloon (Fig. 9.3) that corresponds to the narrowed segment and disappears as the lesion is successfully dilated. Balloons capable of withstanding inflation pressures as high as 15 atm are available for lesions that are resistant to lower inflation pressures.

After dilatation, arterial pressure is measured above and below the lesion so that the success of the procedure can be objectively assessed. A repeat arteriogram may be performed at this time to demonstrate the dilated segment and make sure that no peripheral emboli are present. Unless bleeding occurs, protamine is not given to counter the heparin effect at the end of the procedure.

Although the exact mechanism of balloon angioplasty is still being debated, it seems that several different factors are involved, including plaque remodeling, irreversible overstretching of the muscular wall of the media, and tearing of the intima both at the junction of the plaque and the

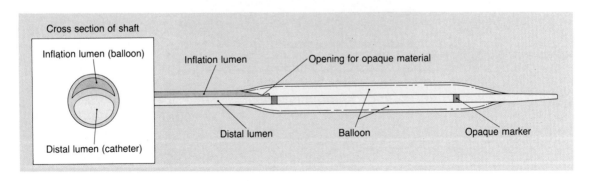

Fig. 9.1 Structure of an angioplasty catheter.

normal vessel wall and opposite the plaque (Fig. 9.4). Expression of the liquid elements of the plaque and compaction of the plaque are minimal, if they occur at all. Because balloon angioplasty is, in effect, a controlled injury to the vessel wall, antiplatelet agents are given before and after the procedure to minimize platelet deposition and thrombosis at the site of intimal disruption.

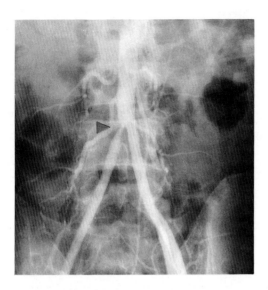

Fig. 9.2 Iliac artery angioplasty. *An arteriogram shows a high-grade stenosis (arrow), extending for a length of 2.5 cm, at the origin of the right common iliac artery. There is a pressure gradient of 10 mm Hg across the stenosis. The balloon catheter should be inflated to a diameter equal to that of the uninvolved artery just distal to the stenosis.*

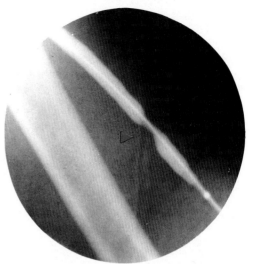

Fig. 9.3 Balloon "waist." *The "waist" (arrow) in the inflated angioplasty balloon corresponds to the site of stenosis in the blood vessel. This "waist" disappears with successful dilatation of the blood vessel.*

Fig. 9.4 Findings after iliac artery angioplasty. *After PTA of the artery shown in Fig. 9.2, contrast material (arrows) is seen within the tear in the arterial wall, a frequent finding after a successful angioplasty.*

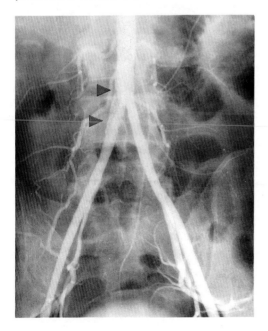

RESULTS

The results of transluminal balloon angioplasty depend primarily on the etiology of the lesion, on which vessel is being dilated, and on whether stenosis or occlusion is present. In general, dilatation of multiple lesions, long-segment lesions, and occlusions is less likely to be successful than dilatation of a single short-segment lesion.

Iliac and Superficial Femoral Arteries

In several recent series, the five-year patency rate after iliac artery angioplasty is approximately 90 percent, which is about the same as the five-year patency rate after surgery. The two- to five-year patency rates reported after superficial femoral artery angioplasty range from 40 to 80 percent. Although these rates are generally lower than those reported for femoral-popliteal vein bypass grafts, they are similar to those reported for bypass grafts with prosthetic materials. Late occlusion of the superficial femoral artery after PTA is due in part to progression of disease in areas of the artery that have not been dilated.

Renal Arteries

The patency rate after renal artery angioplasty is similar to that observed after iliac artery angio-

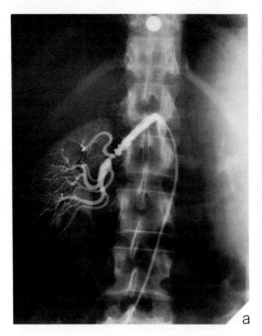

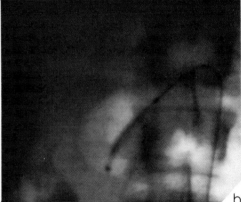

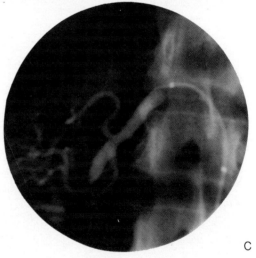

Fig. 9.5 Renal artery angioplasty in fibromuscular disease. *Renal venous blood samples revealed an elevated renin level on the right in this 38-year-old hypertensive patient.* **a** *A selective right renal arteriogram demonstrates fibromuscular disease of the right renal artery.* **b** *The angioplasty catheter, with its balloon inflated, traverses the stenotic segment of the renal artery.* **c** *Following deflation of the balloon, an arteriogram obtained via the angioplasty catheter shows a nearly normal lumen.*

plasty. The results of renal artery angioplasty are significantly affected by the etiology and location of the lesion. The best results have been achieved in patients with fibromuscular disease (Fig. 9.5): About 75 percent of these patients manifest reduced systemic blood pressure, and more than 50 percent no longer require antihypertensive medication. Success rates are lower for atherosclerotic lesions of the renal artery (Fig. 9.6). The best results have been achieved in patients with unilateral stenosis that does not involve the ostium: blood pressure is lowered in 60 to 70 percent of subjects, and about 40 percent no longer require antihypertensive medication. The success rate for lesions involving the ostium is significantly lower.

Other Arteries

The results of dilatation of the abdominal aorta, the subclavian arteries, the carotid arteries, the veretebral arteries, and the visceral arteries cannot be accurately analyzed, because of the small number of procedures and the lack of long-term followup.

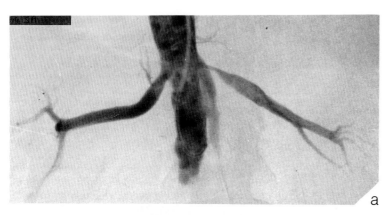

a

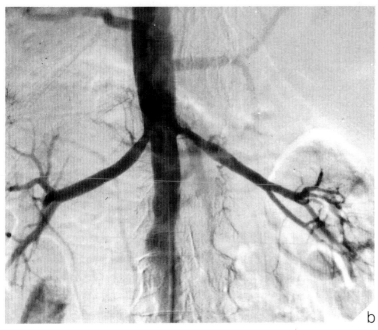

b

Fig. 9.6 Renal artery angioplasty. *a* An aortogram shows atherosclerotic narrowing at the origin of the left renal artery without significant associated aortic disease. *b* After angioplasty, the luminal diameter has increased by more than 50 percent, and the gradient measured across the lesion has been abolished.

COMPLICATIONS

The complications of transluminal angioplasty are few and minor. The most common complication is hematoma at the puncture site (Fig. 9.7). Arterial thrombosis, either at the site of dilatation or at the arterial puncture site, is infrequent. Peripheral embolization occurs in as many as 5 percent of patients; it usually is clinically insignificant. Angioplasty of iliac artery occlusions appears to carry a higher risk of peripheral embolization than angioplasty of occlusions at other sites. Arterial rupture is rare and is sometimes associated with inadvertent balloon rupture (Fig. 9.8).

Subintimal passage of the guidewire during attempts to transverse a high-grade obstruction is not uncommon. It seldom leads to serious sequelae during angioplasty of the iliac or superficial femoral arteries; however, in a peripheral vessel, such as the popliteal or tibial artery, it can result in loss of a limb. Consequently, angioplasty of the popliteal or tibial arteries should be undertaken only in patients with severe ischemia, rest pain, or threatened limb loss.

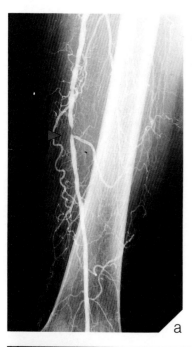
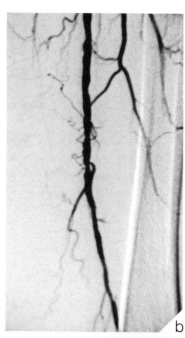

a

b

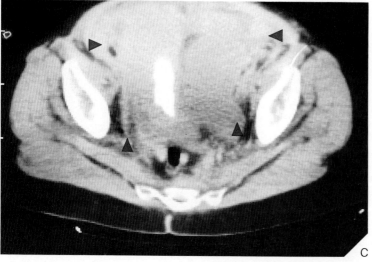

c

Fig. 9.7 Superficial femoral artery angioplasty complicated by pelvic hematoma. *a* An arteriogram shows an isolated short-segment stenosis (arrow) *in the superficial femoral artery at the level of the adductor canal. Although the lumen was almost completely occluded, the stenotic segment was easily traversed with a straight floppy guidewire introduced via the common femoral artery.* ***b*** *An arteriogram obtained after angioplasty shows that the lumen has been reestablished. The occlusion of the small collateral vessel in the region of the angioplasty is of no clinical consequence.* ***c*** *Heparin administered during the angioplasty was not reversed with protamine at the end of the procedure. One hour after the angioplasty, after an episode of coughing, the patient experienced sharp left-sided pelvic pain. Her hemoglobin level fell by 2 g/dL in the next few hours. An emergency CT scan documented a self-limited but significant pelvic hemorrhage (arrows) that was secondary to leakage at the arterial puncture site.*

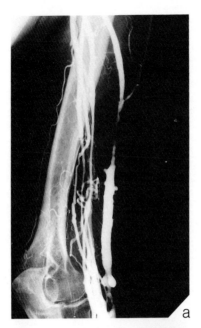

a

Fig. 9.8 Rupture of hemodialysis fistula during angioplasty. *a* An arteriogram shows a long narrowed segment in the arterialized efferent ("out") vein of a surgically created radial artery/radial vein hemodialysis fistula.
b Rupture of the angioplasty catheter balloon during PTA results in the formation of a false aneurysm (arrow) at the angioplasty site.

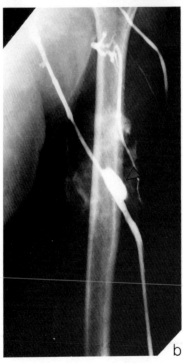

b

CHAPTER TEN

Percutaneous Nephrostomy

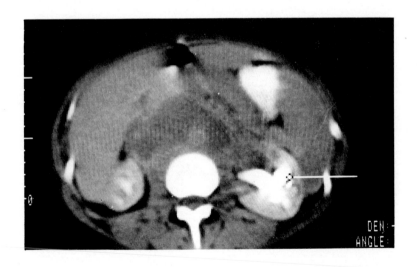

Percutaneous nephrostomy is a therapeutic procedure for decompression of obstructed urinary collecting systems. It also allows access to the urinary system for percutaneous removal or dissolution of renal or ureteral stones, ureteral stenting, nephroscopy, ureteroscopy, and endoscopic resection.

TECHNIQUE

The technique used for percutaneous nephrostomy varies according to the indication for the procedure. If percutaneous nephrostomy is being performed to relieve obstruction, it is best done under the guidance of real-time ultrasound. With the patient mildly sedated, the skin and needle tract are infiltrated with a local anesthetic. A dilated posterior calyx is identified sonographically and punctured with a 20-gauge needle. A .018-in. guidewire is then passed through the needle into the renal collecting system. The nephrostomy tract is enlarged (Fig. 10.1) by the insertion of progressively larger dilators and guidewires until an 8-French nephrostomy catheter can be introduced into the renal pelvis (Fig. 10.2). Care must be taken to allow the guidewire sufficient purchase within the collecting system that it is not displaced during passage of the dilators and the nephrostomy catheter. Inadvertent puncture of the spleen, liver, colon, or lung can be avoided by careful planning of the access route (Fig. 10.3).

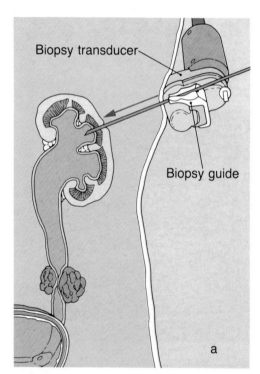

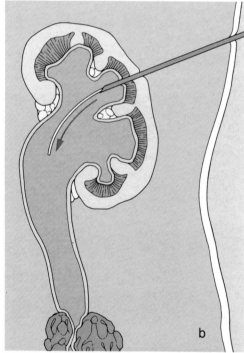

Fig. 10.1 Technique for percutaneous nephrostomy. *a Under continuous real-time ultrasound guidance, a posterior calyx is punctured with a 20-gauge needle. **b** Through this needle, a .018-in. stiff guidewire is passed distally into the dilated renal pelvis or ureter. **c** A one-step conversion catheter is passed over the guidewire. **d** A .035-in. guidewire is passed through the side port of the conversion catheter into the renal pelvis. **e** In succession, 6-, 7-, and 8-French dilators are passed over the guidewire. **f** An 8-French nephrostomy catheter is then passed over the guidewire and left in the renal pelvis.*

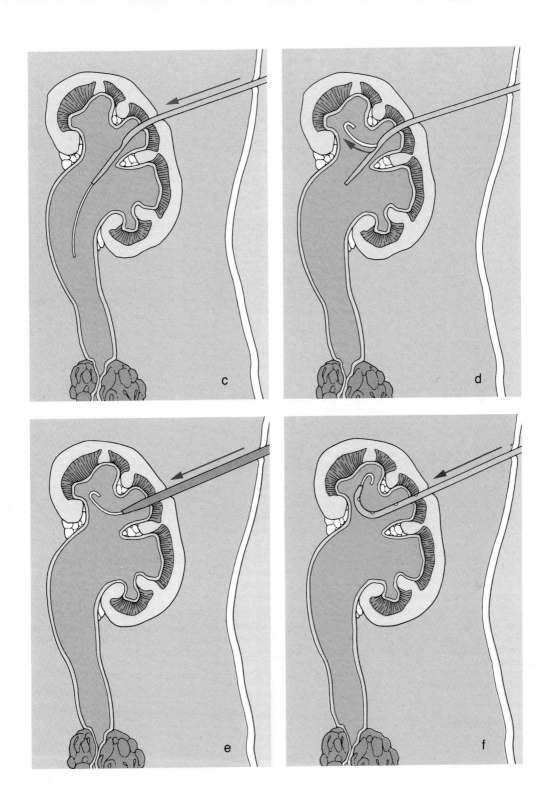

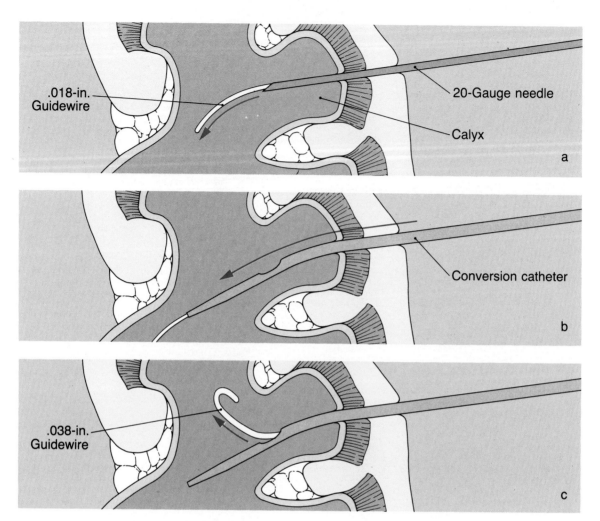

Fig. 10.2 One-step conversion system. *Several systems are available for introduction of .038-in. guidewires after puncture with 20-gauge needles that accept only .018-in. guidewires. The system illustrated here is ideal for procedures that require access to the renal collecting system or biliary tract.* **a** *After puncture of the calyx or duct with a 20-gauge needle, a .018-in. guidewire is passed through the needle and advanced into the system. The end of the guidewire is flexible, but the rest of the wire is stiff.* **b** *A conversion catheter with a .018-in. end hole and a more proximal .038-in. side hole is passed over the guidewire. When the catheter is in the desired space, the .018-in. wire is removed and replaced with a .038-in. wire.* **c** *Because of the rapid tapering of the catheter tip, the .038-in. guidewire must exit through the side hole.*

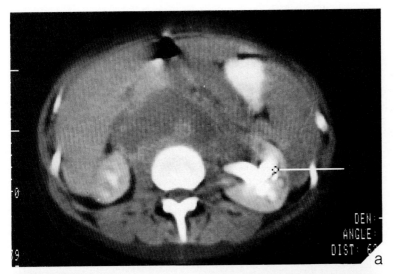

Fig. 10.3 Anatomic considerations for percutaneous nephrostomy. *CT scans at the level of the kidneys demonstrate midline retroperitoneal adenopathy and bilateral hydronephrosis.*
a Puncture of the upper pole calyces of the left kidney with too anterior an approach would inadvertently puncture the spleen.
b Puncture of a lower pole calyx with too anterior an approach would lead to puncture of the descending colon. c This can be avoided by introducing the needle at the posterior axillary line and angling it anteriorly.

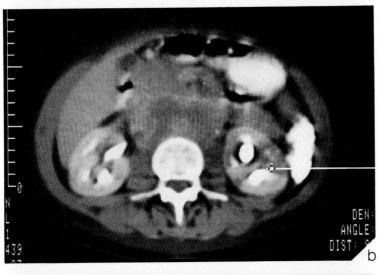

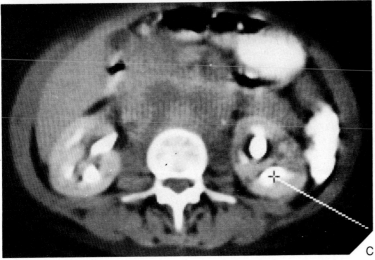

CLINICAL APPLICATIONS

Relief of Obstruction

Percutaneous nephrostomy is a simple, rapid, and safe method for decompressing an obstructed kidney. In a patient with renal failure secondary to bilateral ureteral obstruction whose renal function is otherwise normal, decompression of one kidney will reverse the renal failure. A pigtail catheter left in the renal pelvis (Fig. 10.4) provides external drainage of the obstructed kidney. An alternative technique is to manipulate a guidewire beyond the point of obstruction, then advance a drainage catheter over the guidewire into the bladder. The drainage catheter is positioned so that the side holes lie above and below the obstruction; this placement allows internal drainage of urine into the bladder while maintaining external access (Fig. 10.5). Another approach, which leaves the patient with no external appliances, is to advance a double-pigtail internal stent over a guidewire, positioning one pigtail in the renal pelvis and the other in the urinary bladder (Fig. 10.6). Percutaneous stent placement eliminates the need for general anesthesia and is frequently more successful at relieving obstruction than is endoscopic transvesical stent placement; moreover, it keeps the obstructed collecting system from being contaminated by bacteria from the urethra and bladder, a potential hazard of endoscopic retrograde techniques (Fig. 10.7).

Stenting and balloon dilatation followed by stenting are gaining favor in the management of ureteral strictures. Surgery remains the primary treatment for congenital ureteropelvic junction obstruction; however, surgical failures often can be successfully managed by balloon dilatation and stenting of the strictured segment.

Percutaneous Stone Removal

Access to renal calculi depends on puncturing the renal collecting system through the proper calyx. To approach stones in the renal pelvis, all that is necessary is to puncture any posterior calyx from the posterior axillary line. To approach intracalyceal calculi, however, it is necessary to puncture the calyx containing the stone. Since precise localization of the calyces is essential, these nephrostomies must be performed under fluoroscopic guidance. The collecting system can be opacified by intravenous injection, retrograde injection of the ureter (via a ureteral catheter), or percutaneous injection (in which case a second percutaneous puncture is needed to enter the proper calyx so that the stone can be removed). Carbon dioxide or air, introduced into the collecting system with the patient prone, can be used to identify the posterior calyces.

Once the appropriate calyx has been entered, a guidewire is passed through the calyx and the renal pelvis and advanced down the ureter to the level of the urinary bladder. Over this guidewire is placed a sheath, through which additional guidewires, which serve as "safety" wires in the event that the first guidewire is dislodged from the collecting system, are introduced. Progressively larger fascial dilators, or balloon dilatation catheters in conjunction with fascial dilators, are inserted until a 30- to 32-French tract is created. A 32-French sheath is advanced over the last fascial dilator into the collecting system (Fig. 10.8). An endoscope is introduced through this sheath, and stones are fragmented under direct endoscopic control. Stones 18 mm or less in diameter may be retrieved with a stone basket under fluoroscopic control. Although the initial nephrostomy can be performed with the patient under local anesthesia, dilatation of the tract and stone fragmentation necessitate general anesthesia.

COMPLICATIONS

Percutaneous nephrostomy performed to relieve obstruction is rarely associated with complications; those most often observed are hemorrhage and urine extravasation. Although bleeding commonly accompanies percutaneous nephrostomy, it almost always is self-limited, and it rarely requires intervention. Extravasation of urine due to perforation of the collecting system during guidewire or catheter manipulation is treated by means of the nephrostomy tube and seldom gives rise to significant morbidity.

Nephrostomy procedures performed to remove renal stones have a higher complication rate than drainage procedures do. Most of the complications are accounted for by hemorrhage (which may necessitate blood transfusion or surgery) and perforation of the collecting system by guidewires or instruments. Penetration of bowel or solid viscera is also a potential complication.

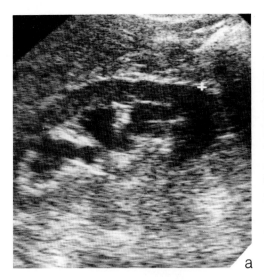

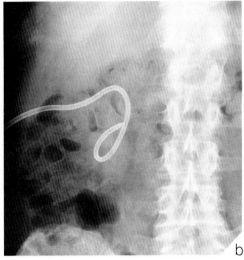

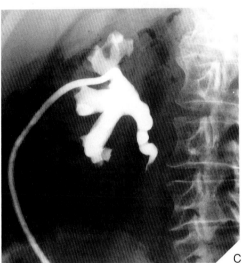

Fig. 10.4 Percutaneous nephrostomy.
a Longitudinal ultrasonogram of the right kidney in a patient with metastatic prostate carcinoma demonstrates moderate hydronephrosis secondary to extensive retroperitoneal adenopathy. A percutaneous nephrostomy was placed under sonographic and fluoroscopic control using the technique illustrated in Fig. 10.1. *b* A plain film taken at the end of the procedure shows an 8-French pigtail nephrostomy catheter in place. *c* Injection through the nephrostomy catheter reveals complete obstruction of the proximal ureter by enlarged retroperitoneal lymph nodes.

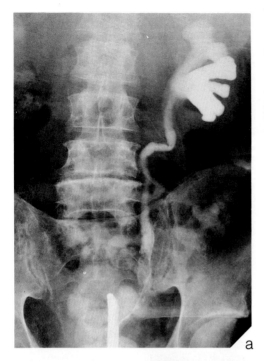

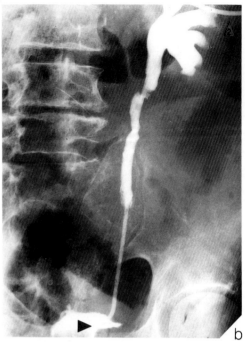

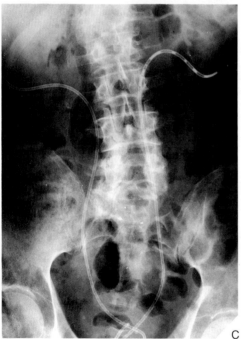

Fig. 10.5 Ureteral stenting using a catheter with an external port. *a* A retrograde pyelogram from a 70-year-old patient with a solitary left kidney and renal failure as a result of obstructive uropathy shows a primary ureteral tumor that completely obstructs the left ureter. After an unsuccessful attempt at retrograde stent placement, antegrade stent placement was accomplished under sonographic and fluoroscopic guidance. *b* An antegrade contrast injection shows the tip of the stent (arrow 1) beyond the ureteral lesion. Positioning of the side holes above the lesion allows urine to drain from the obstructed ureter into the bladder. The external port (arrow 2) provides a route for irrigation and can be used to replace the catheter if it becomes occluded. *c* Bilateral ureteral stents with external ports have been placed in this patient, a woman with bilateral ureteral obstruction due to endometrial carcinoma.

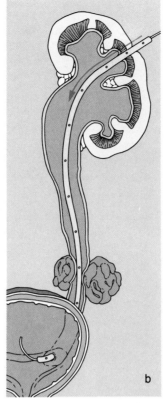
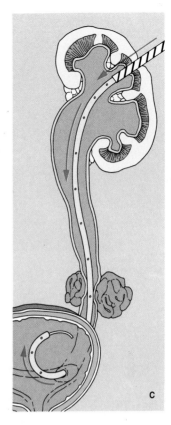
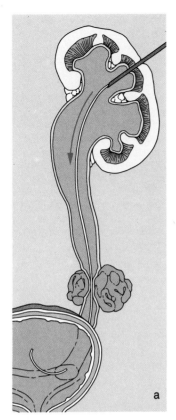
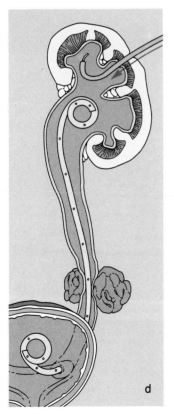

Fig. 10.6 Technique for antegrade stent placement. *a After access to the renal collecting system is gained in the standard fashion, a straight angiographic guidewire or torque wire is passed through the region of ureteral obstruction and into the bladder. **b** After the tract has been dilated to the desired size, a double-pigtail catheter is straightened and passed over the guidewire. **c** The pigtail catheter is advanced by a "pusher" catheter until one end is in the urinary bladder and the other is in the renal pelvis. **d** The guidewire is then withdrawn into the renal pelvis. When the guidewire is removed from the catheter, the pigtail catheter acquires its desired shape. A nephrostomy catheter is advanced over the guidewire into the renal pelvis and is left in place until the internal stent is shown to be functioning properly.*

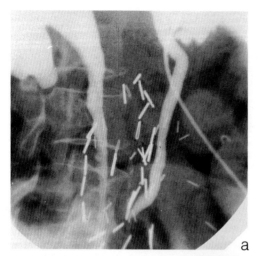

a

Fig. 10.7 Percutaneous internal stent placement. *A woman with advanced cervical carcinoma presented with renal failure due to obstructive uropathy. Both ureters had previously been diverted into an ileal conduit.*
***a** Antegrade pyelography via percutaneous nephrostomy catheters demonstrates bilateral ureteral obstruction secondary to retroperitoneal adenopathy. Percutaneous antegrade stenting was performed. **b** On the left, an internal stent has been advanced into the ileal conduit (arrows 1). An internal double-pigtail stent is in place on the right; one end is in the renal pelvis, the other in the ileal conduit (arrows 2). A nephrostomy catheter (arrow 3) has been placed alongside the internal stent on the left; it will remain in place until satisfactory function of the stent is assured (about 48 hours).*

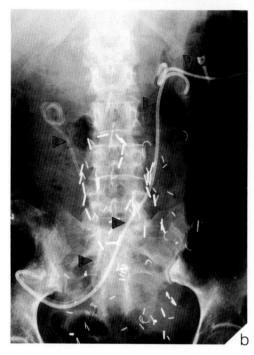

b

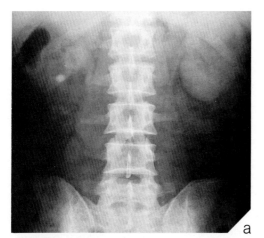

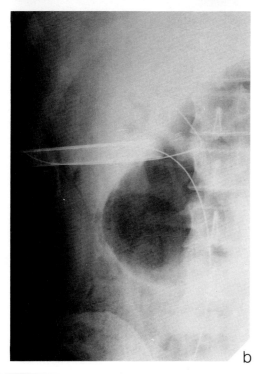

Fig. 10.8 Percutaneous renal stone removal.
a An intravenous urogram demonstrates a large calculus in a right lower pole calyx. After percutaneous access to the calyx containing the calculus was achieved, a tract was dilated to 34 French. b The sheath through which the endoscope will be introduced has been advanced into the tract and positioned adjacent to the renal calculus. Note the "safety" wires in the renal pelvis and ureter.

*I*nterventional Procedures in the Biliary Tract

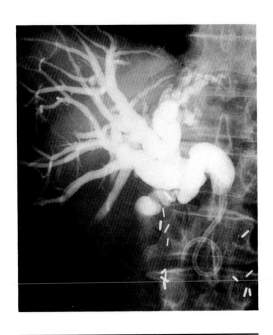

The first example of radiologic intervention in the biliary system was the removal of retained common bile duct stones through the tracts of surgically placed T-tubes. Procedures such as percutaneous biliary bypass, stenting and dilatation of bile ducts narrowed by tumor or inflammatory changes, and percutaneous removal of bile duct stones are natural extensions of percutaneous transhepatic cholangiography. To all of these procedures there exist surgical and gastroenterologic alternatives; consequently, a multidisciplinary approach is crucial for ensuring selection of the procedure best suited to the patient's overall needs.

REMOVAL OF RETAINED BILE DUCT STONES

Bile duct stones retained after surgery are easily removed through the previously established T-tube tract. The procedure is generally performed four to six weeks after bile duct exploration, by which time a fibrous tract has formed around the T-tube. The procedure has had a success rate of more than 95 percent in experienced hands.

Technique

Bile duct stone removal is usually performed on an outpatient basis with the patient under moder-ate sedation and local anesthesia (Fig. 11.1). A guidewire is inserted through the T-tube into the bile duct and advanced to the region of the retained common bile duct or hepatic duct stone. A Teflon catheter is passed over the guidewire and advanced beyond the stone. The guidewire is then removed, and a stone basket is introduced into the catheter. As the basket is held in place, the catheter is withdrawn far enough to allow the basket to open. Both the catheter and the basket are then withdrawn until the basket engages the stone. (It is often necessary to rotate the basket.) If the basket and the stone move synchronously upon manipulation, the stone is engaged in the basket. The catheter is then advanced toward the basket to lock the stone in place. The T-tube, the catheter, and the basket with the stone are then withdrawn as a unit. At the end of the procedure, a repeat cholangiogram is obtained to verify that all the stones have been removed.

If the initial attempt at stone retrieval is unsuccessful, a guidewire, followed by a catheter and a basket, can be reinserted through the established tract and the procedure repeated. If necessary, the T-tube can be replaced.

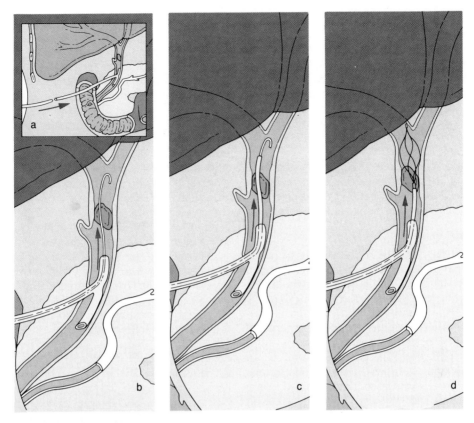

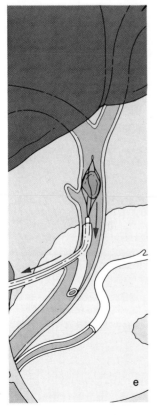

Fig. 11.1 Biliary stone removal through a T-tube. *a* A common hepatic duct stone is located proximal to a surgi-cally placed T-tube. *b* A guidewire inserted through the T-tube is passed proximal to the stone. *c* A catheter is placed over the guidewire and advanced beyond the stone. *d* The guidewire is removed, and a stone basket is inserted into the catheter. The catheter is pulled back far enough to allow the basket to open. *e* The basket is with-drawn, engaging the stone. Once the stone is engaged in the basket, the basket (containing the stone) and the T-tube are removed as one from the patient.

PERCUTANEOUS BILIARY BYPASS

Percutaneous biliary bypass allows external or internal drainage of bile ducts obstructed by tumors, strictures, or stones. It can offer palliation to patients who are not candidates for surgery because of poor general health or a poor prognosis. Some lesions that are difficult to approach surgically (e.g., porta hepatis metastases or intrahepatic duct obstruction) are readily bypassed with percutaneous techniques.

Percutaneous access to the biliary system also provides a method of percutaneous stone removal, percutaneous dilatation of obstructed bile ducts, and percutaneous biopsy of the biliary tract.

Technique

To minimize the risk of biliary sepsis, the patient is placed on parenteral antibiotic therapy prior to the procedure. The procedure is performed with the patient under local anesthesia and moderately sedated. A right lateral 11th or 12th intercostal or subcostal approach is employed for entering a right hepatic duct, an anterior approach for entering a left hepatic duct. The first step is to obtain a fine-needle percutaneous transhepatic cholangiogram in order to visualize the obstructed biliary system. When the intrahepatic ducts are well opacified, a peripheral hepatic duct directly aligned with the common bile duct is punctured with an 18- or 20-gauge needle under fluoroscopic control (Fig. 11.2). An extrinsic deformity of the duct caused by the approach of the needle disappears once the needle enters the lumen. A guidewire (.018 to .038 mm, depending on needle size) is then introduced through the needle and advanced to the point of obstruction. Dilators and catheters are passed over the guidewire and advanced as far distally as possible to provide maximum guidewire purchase within the system. Straight floppy guidewires, or stiffer steerable torque wires that can be directed through the lesion, are used to bypass the obstruction, after which the duct can be dilated and the catheter placed (Fig. 11.3).

The drainage catheter has multiple side holes, which are positioned above and below the lesion. The pigtail end is placed In the duodenum for internal drainage, and the external hub is connected to a bile bag for external drainage (Fig. 11.4). After a short initial period of external drainage, the external port is occluded, and internal drainage is established. Biliary bypass can be performed through either the right or the left hepatic ducts (Figs. 11.5, 11.6). Ultrasonic guidance may facilitate puncture of left hepatic ducts.

Alternatively, an internal stent can be placed to provide internal drainage, without an external appliance for external drainage (Fig. 11.7a, b). Since no external port is available for catheter exchange, a repeat bypass procedure must be performed if obstruction occurs (Fig. 11.7c).

Results and Complications

Percutaneous biliary bypass techniques successfully establish external drainage in more than 90 percent of patients and internal drainage in approximately 75 to 80 percent. Early complications include hemorrhage from the liver puncture and bile leak. Intermediate and late complications are generally associated with the indwelling catheter; they include catheter dislodgment, occlusion, sepsis (see Fig. 11.6b), and hemorrhage into the biliary tract. Although catheter-related complications are usually minor, they occur in the majority of patients, and they must be taken into account whenever a percutaneous bypass procedure is being contemplated.

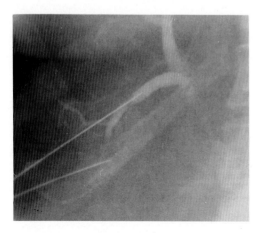

Fig. 11.2 Double puncture. *Opacification of the right hepatic ducts was obtained by injecting contrast material though the lower needle. Under direct visualization, a right hepatic duct in good alignment with the common hepatic duct was then punctured with the upper needle.*

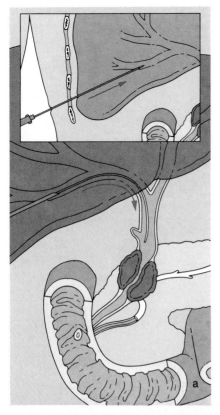

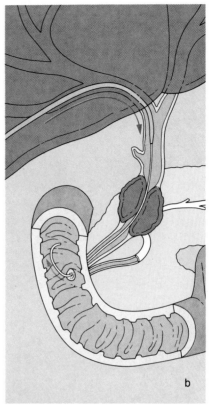

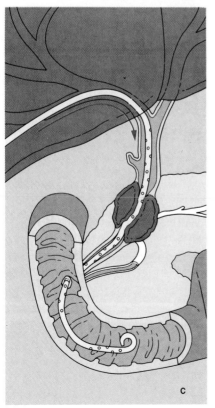

Fig. 11.3 Percutaneous biliary bypass. *a* After puncture of a right hepatic duct with an 18- or 20-gauge needle, a guidewire is passed through the lumen of the needle and advanced into the obstructed system. *b* A catheter is passed over the guidewire, and guidewire and catheter are manipulated into the duodenum. *c* After dilatation of the tract, an 8-French biliary drainage catheter is passed into the obstructed system. The side holes of the catheter are positioned over and below the level of the obstruction, and the pigtail end is placed in the duodenum.

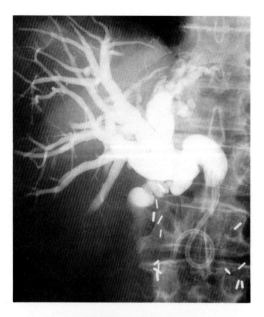

Fig. 11.4 Successful percutaneous biliary bypass. *After a successful procedure, the pigtail end of the drainage catheter is coiled in the duodenum.*

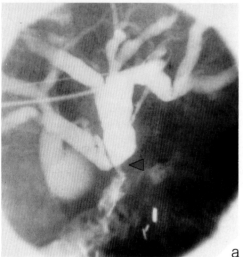

a

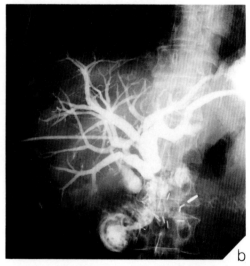

b

Fig. 11.5 Percutaneous biliary bypass. *This patient developed increasing jaundice one year after undergoing a choledochojejunostomy for relief of biliary obstruction caused by a carcinoma of the head of the pancreas. **a** Diagnostic cholangiography demonstrates narrowing due to the tumor (arrow) at the site of the choledo-chojejunal anastomosis. **b** After a successful bypass, a drainage catheter traverses the right and common hepatic ducts. The tip of the catheter is in the proximal jejunum, and there is good flow of contrast material from the bile ducts into the jejunum.*

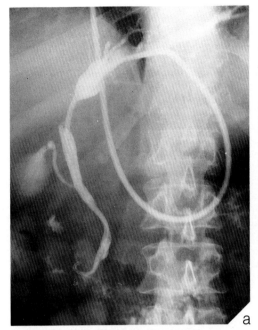

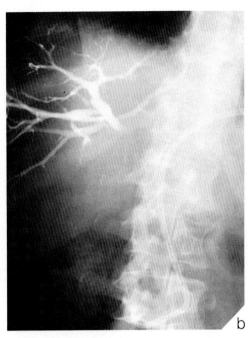

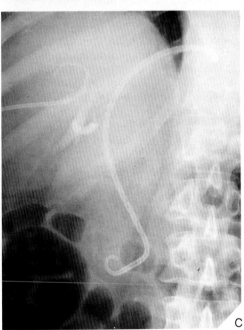

Fig. 11.6 Percutaneous biliary bypass. *In this patient, bypass of a metastasis obstructing the right and common hepatic ducts at the porta hepatis was accomplished via the left hepatic duct system. **a** A cholangiogram performed through the bypass catheter shows opacification of the distal hepatic and common bile ducts with flow of contrast material into the duodenum. There is no opacification of the right hepatic duct system. **b** One month later, the patient returned with sepsis. A percutaneous transhepatic cholangiogram shows isolation of the right hepatic ducts, which presumably became infected from the indwelling left hepatic duct catheter. **c** A pigtail catheter has been placed for external drainage of the right hepatic ducts.*

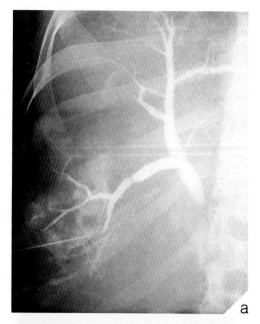

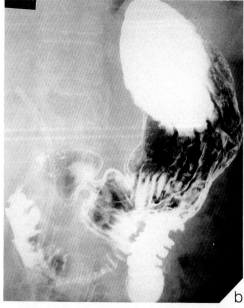

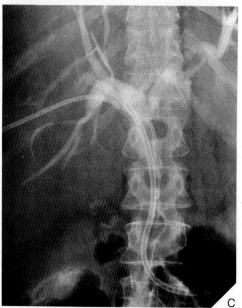

Fig. 11.7 Percutaneous biliary bypass with stent. *a Diagnostic cholangiography demonstrates obstruction of the common bile duct due to carcinoma of the pancreas. b An upper gastrointestinal series after percutaneous placement of an internal biliary stent shows the tip of the stent in the transverse duodenum. One year later, the patient developed progressive jaundice due to obstruction of the stent. Attempts at endoscopic stent replacement were unsuccessful, and the patient underwent a repeat percutaneous biliary bypass procedure with placement of an internal/external drainage catheter. c A percutaneous cholangiogram obtained after the second bypass procedure shows the drainage catheter alongside the nonfunctioning stent. The catheter tip is in the duodenum.*

PERCUTANEOUS CHOLECYSTOSTOMY

Percutaneous cholecystostomy is the radiologic alternative to surgical cholecystostomy: It decompresses the gallbladder in patients with obstruction of the cystic duct. Percutaneous cholecystostomy is particularly useful in patients with acalculous cholecystitis, who frequently are poor surgical candidates. This procedure has in fact been used as the primary treatment in such cases (Fig. 11.8); the best results are obtained if it is performed early in the course of the disease. It should be remembered that patients with gangrenous gallbladders should not be treated with percutaneous techniques.

Because proper patient selection is crucial, sophisticated imaging and a meticulous clinical assessment are essential for identifying suitable candidates for percutaneous cholecystostomy.

Technique

The technique used to carry out percutaneous (transhepatic) cholecystostomy is similar to that used to carry out other percutaneous drainage procedures. The procedure should be done under the guidance either of CT or (preferably) of ultrasound. The drainage catheter is introduced either by the Seldinger technique (i.e., over a guidewire) or by direct puncture of the gallbladder with a one-step drainage catheter. The one-step approach may prevent significant vagal reactions, an occasional sequela of the Seldinger technique. A bile specimen is obtained for laboratory studies; a Gram stain may establish the diagnosis of acute cholecystitis in a patient in whom the diagnosis is in doubt.

The cholecystostomy tube is usually left in place until the patient becomes asymptomatic and contrast injection demonstrates patency of the cystic duct. If cholecystectomy is not planned, the cholecystostomy tube is removed once patency of the cystic duct is demonstrated. If cholecystectomy is planned, the drainage tube is left in place until the time of surgery.

Complications

The complications of percutaneous cholecystostomy include vagal reactions (bradycardia, hypotension, and asystole), gallbladder perforation, and bile sepsis. Inadvertent gallbladder perforation during tube placement can be prevented by placement of the cholecystostomy drainage tube.

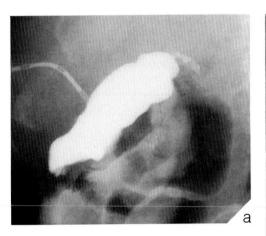

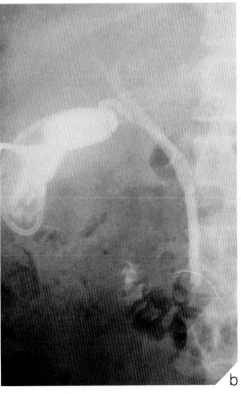

Fig. 11.8 Percutaneous cholecystostomy. *In this patient, percutaneous cholecystostomy was performed under ultrasound guidance to treat acalculous cholecystitis.* **a** *Injection through the drainage catheter demonstrates cystic duct obstruction.* **b** *After the resolution of the acute episode of cholecystitis, injection through the drainage catheter demonstrates patency of the cystic duct with opacification of the common bile duct. The cholecystostomy catheter was removed, and the patient required no further therapy.*

Arterial Infusion and Embolization Procedures

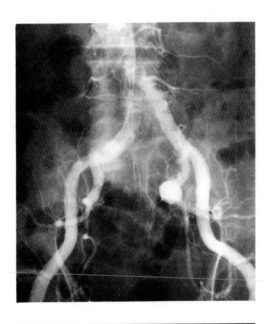

By means of angiographic techniques, the interventional radiologist can gain access to most of the body's organs via the vascular system. Transvascular therapeutic procedures include delivery of materials to produce vascular occlusion, superselective administration of chemotherapeutic and pharmacologic agents, and intravascular placement of various mechanical devices.

VASCULAR OCCLUSIVE PROCEDURES

Angiographic methods are ideally suited to creating a temporary or permanent vascular occlusion (for example, to control hemorrhage, infarct a tumor, or treat a vascular malformation or aneurysm). Vascular occlusion can be produced either in large vessels or in peripheral vascular beds. The size of the vessel to be occluded is determined by particle size and by the physical properties of the occlusive agent.

Materials

The materials used in the creation of vascular occlusions include autologous products, such as blood clot, muscle, or dura; absorbable products, such as surgical gelatin sponge (Gelfoam) and oxidized cellulose (Oxycel); nonabsorbable products, such as polyvinyl alcohol, silicone spheres, detachable balloons, steel coils, and polymers (e.g., isobutyl-2-cyanoacrylate); and absolute alcohol. Electrocoagulation, which does not entail the use of introduced material, is used in a small percentage of cases.

Which material is chosen depends on its availability and on the indication for vascular occlusion. Blood clot is readily available, but it provides only short-term occlusion, since the clot is quickly lysed by the body's fibrinolytic system. Gelfoam is readily available and can be prepared in sizes ranging from powder to large fragments. Although Gelfoam is eventually absorbed, it provides occlusion for a period of several weeks. Polymers provide permanent occlusion, but are not available for general usage. Polyvinyl alcohol is a nonabsorbable particulate material that comes in a variety of sizes and is easily delivered through angiographic catheters. Absolute alcohol is readily available and is easily injected through very small catheters or open guidewires; it provides permanent vascular occlusion and can be delivered distally into the vascular bed. Mechanical devices such as Gianturco coils are very useful for occluding large vessels.

The size of the particle determines the level of vascular occlusion. To infarct a vascular malformation or tumor, and prevent the development of a collateral blood supply, it is necessary to occlude the most distal vascular bed; in such cases, small particles, absolute alcohol, or polymers are used. To minimize the risk of tissue necrosis in treating arterial bleeding, it is necessary to embolize slightly larger arteries. Once hemostasis is attained, the most distal vascular bed will be reperfused by collaterals.

Gastrointestinal Hemorrhage

Interventional radiologists are frequently consulted in the diagnosis and treatment of gastrointestinal hemorrhage. In patients with upper gastrointestinal hemorrhage, endoscopy is employed for diagnosis and angiography reserved for treatment. Patients with bleeding esophageal varices are usually treated with systemic infusion of vasopressin through a peripheral vein; selective infusion of vasopressin into the superior mesenteric artery has not proved more effective than peripheral infusion. Endoscopic sclerosis of esophageal varices has received a great deal of attention recently, but transportal variceal occlusion with alcohol, coils, or particulate material (after selective catheterization of the coronary vein and other collaterals) can provide excellent short-term management of variceal hemorrhage (Fig. 12.1). Unfortunately, however, this procedure offers poor long-term control of hemorrhage, particularly in Child's class B and C patients.

Patients with diffusely bleeding gastritis or Mallory-Weiss tears are effectively treated with either vasopressin infusion or embolization of the left gastric artery. Hemorrhage from gastric and duodenal ulcers is a more difficult problem; vasopressin treatment is successful in only 50 percent of cases, and embolization in approximately 75 percent. Because hemorrhage from a peptic ulcer is frequently an indication for surgical intervention, embolization should be reserved for patients who are poor surgical risks.

Arterial embolization can be performed safely throughout the upper gastrointestinal tract, provided that a pathway for collateral blood flow is available. Patients with severe atherosclerotic disease and those who have undergone extensive upper gastrointestinal surgery are at higher risk for bowel infarction after embolization. In these subjects, embolization should be performed with extreme caution, if at all. In patients undergoing embolization of the arteries that supply the liver, patency of the portal vein should be confirmed.

Small-bowel hemorrhage may be treated either with arterial infusion of vasopressors or with arterial embolization. Embolization of the small bowel carries a greater risk of bowel infarction than upper gastrointestinal embolization.

Diverticular hemorrhage of the colon can be satisfactorily treated by infusion of vasopressin (0.2–0.4 U/min) into the superior or inferior mesenteric artery (Fig. 12.2). Vasopressin infusion controls the hemorrhage in 90 percent of patients; bleeding recurs in fewer than one third, usually soon after the infusion is stopped.

Hemorrhage at Other Sites

Transcatheter embolization is useful in managing hemorrhage secondary to trauma, neoplasm, vascular malformations, and aneurysms. The choice of embolic agent depends on the lesion being treated and on whether the goal is tissue infarction or hemostasis. For tumor infarction (Fig. 12.3), embolization should be carried out at the level of the smallest vessel possible, so that collateral blood supply to tumor vessels is minimized and complete infarction can take place. For pelvic hemorrhage secondary to trauma or neoplasm (Fig. 12.4), the goal is hemostasis and preservation of tissue, which means that particles of larger size must be used. In treating arterial aneurysms, the goal is to thrombose the aneurysm while preserving as much of the peripheral vascular bed as possible; this is best accomplished with large mechanical devices such as the Gianturco coils (Fig. 12.5).

Treatment of Neoplastic Disease

Transvascular embolization effectively decreases or eliminates the vascular supply to a tumor, and therefore can result in a reduction in tumor size. It may be either an adjunct to or a substitute for surgery. Embolization has proved effective in relieving the symptoms of painful tumor masses (e.g., bone metastases); other metastases, especially those secreting vasoactive substances (e.g., carcinoid tumors), also readily respond to arterial embolization. Unfortunately, it has not been conclusively shown that arterial embolization effectively increases long-term survival.

Chemotherapeutic agents may be delivered locally to a tumor bed, which makes it possible to administer larger doses of chemotherapeutic agents to the tumor with fewer systemic side effects (Fig. 12.6). The benefits of this technique must be weighed against the risk of catheter-related complications such as local and distal arterial thrombosis.

Prevention of Pulmonary Thromboembolism

Pulmonary thromboemboli account for a large percentage of deaths in a hospital population. Although heparin administration is a safe and effective method for preventing pulmonary emboli, there are patients in whom it is ineffective or contraindicated. In these persons, placement of the cage-like Kimray–Greenfield filter is effective in preventing pulmonary emboli. The rate of pulmonary embolism after filter placement is 2 percent, which is comparable to that observed in patients who have received adequate anticoagulation therapy.

The filter is placed transvenously after either a surgical cutdown or a percutaneous puncture (Fig. 12.7). An access tract is dilated to permit introduction of the filter carrier. The filter is generally placed just below the renal veins in patients with documented thrombosis of lower-extremity or pelvic veins. Complications related to the use of the Kimray–Greenfield filter are uncommon. Vena caval occlusion occurs in fewer than 5 percent of patients, and lower extremity venous stasis in fewer than 6 percent. Filter migration is not a significant concern.

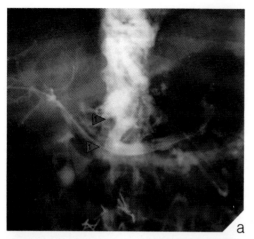

Fig. 12.1 Transhepatic embolization of the coronary vein. *This 41-year-old alcoholic presented with massive hemorrhage from esophageal varices that was refractory to endoscopic sclerotherapy. **a, b** A transhepatic splenoportogram demonstrates a large coronary vein (arrows 1) supplying numerous large esophageal varices (arrows 2). **c** After embolization of the varices with alcohol and Gianturco coils, the hemorrhage stopped. A repeat splenoportogram reveals occlusion of the coronary vein at its origin (arrow). Several coils are seen distally in the occluded coronary vein.*

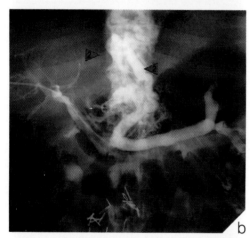

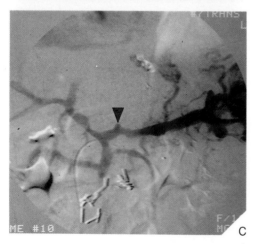

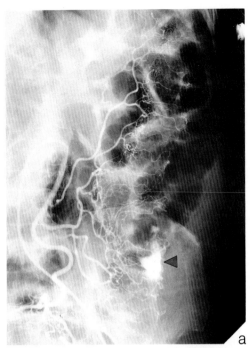

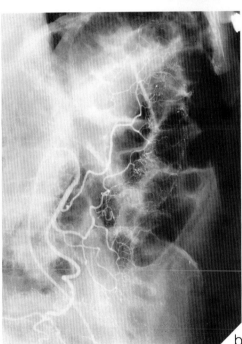

Fig. 12.2 Vasopressin infusion for diverticular hemorrhage. *a Selective injection of the inferior mesenteric artery demonstrates contrast extravasation into the lumen of the colon at the site of a diverticular hemorrhage (arrow). Vasopressin was infused at a rate of 0.2 U/min. b A repeat arteriogram obtained after 20 minutes of vasopressin infusion shows no further bleeding into the diverticulum. Vasopressin was tapered over 24 hours, and the patient had no further bleeding.*

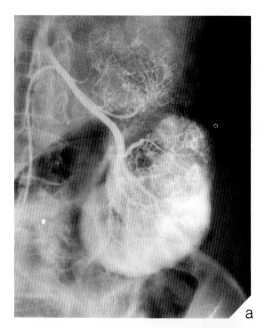

a

Fig. 12.3 Embolization of renal carcinoma.
*a A selective left renal artery arteriogram
reveals a hypervascular hypernephroma.
b Embolization was accomplished with
Gelfoam and several large Gianturco coils.
A repeat arteriogram shows complete occlusion of the left renal artery with three Gianturco
coils in place* (arrows).

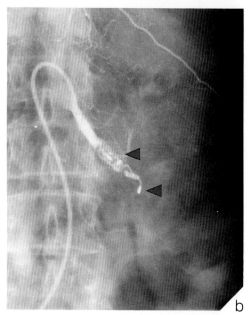

b

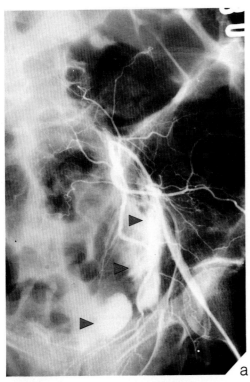

Fig. 12.4 Embolization of the internal iliac artery. *a* Selective injection of the internal iliac artery in a woman with advanced cervical cancer demonstrates extravasation of contrast material (arrows) at the site of a pelvic hemorrhage. *b* After embolization of medial division branches of the internal iliac artery with polyvinyl alcohol particles, all of the medial division branches are occluded. There is no further evidence of bleeding.

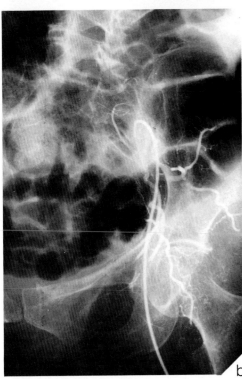

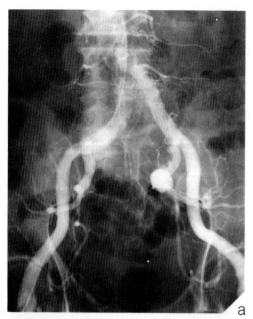

Fig. 12.5 Embolization of an iliac artery aneurysm. *a A distal abdominal aortogram obtained with the catheter at the aortic bifurcation reveals an internal iliac artery aneurysm. b Gelfoam and Gianturco coils were used to occlude the aneurysm. A repeat aortogram shows coils in the aneurysm and one lateral division branch of the internal iliac artery. The aneurysm is no longer seen.*

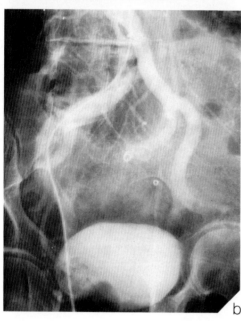

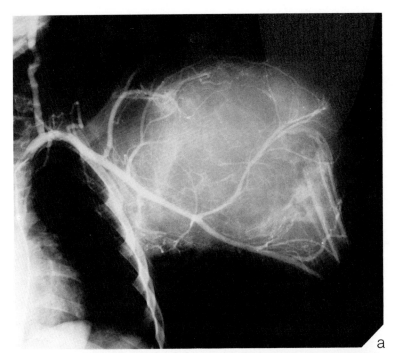

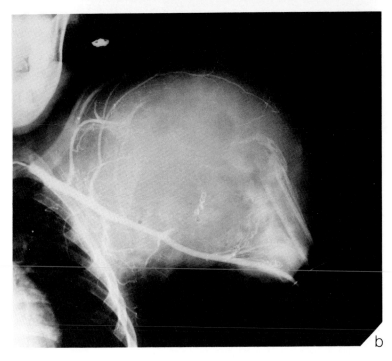

Fig. 12.6 Embolization of osteosarcoma. *a* A left subclavian arteriogram demonstrates tumor neovascularity associated with a large osteosarcoma of the humerus. *b* A repeat arteriogram after embolization with alcohol and Gianturco coils showed that all but one of the major arterial feeders to the tumor have been occluded. Chemotherapeutic agents were then infused via this artery directly into the tumor.

a

b

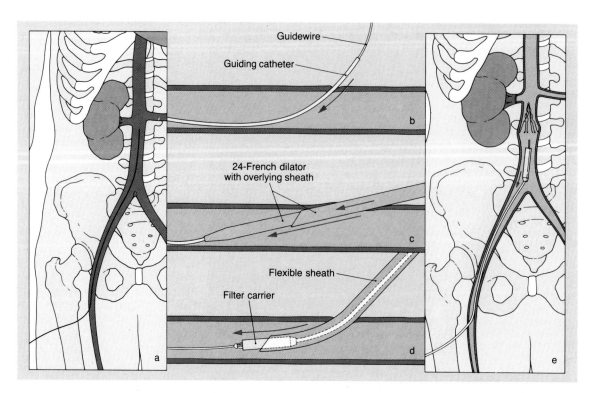

Fig. 12.7 Kimray–Greenfield filter. *a* Upon percutaneous puncture of the femoral vein a guidewire is placed into the vena cava to the level of the renal veins. *b* A guiding catheter is placed over the guidewire. *c* Progressively larger fascial dilators up to 24 French are placed over the guiding catheter to dilate the femoral vein puncture hole to the desired diameter. *d* A flexible sheath of 24–26 French is placed in the femoral vein and through the sheath the Kimray–Greenfield filter and carrier are placed over the guidewire and to a level just immediately below the most inferior renal vein. *e* Following placement of the carrier in correct position, the filter is expelled and carrier, sheath, and wires are removed from the patient.

THROMBOLYTIC THERAPY FOR ARTERIAL THROMBI

Lysis of thrombi in situ is effective in reestablishing blood flow to the peripheral vascular bed. Lysis of thrombi or emboli in a native artery or arterial graft can be accomplished by means of fibrinolytic agents infused locally through a catheter placed in the occluded vessel (Fig. 12.8). Unfortunately, transcatheter thrombolytic therapy is not universally successful: The complication rate can be as high as 50 percent. The complications include local and distant bleeding (Fig. 12.9), thrombosis related to the indwelling catheter, and distal embolization of the lysed clot. Whereas some published reports indicate complete clot lysis in as many as 75 percent of patients, others indicate that the success rate is below 40 percent, with more complications than cures. It is generally agreed that thrombi less than a week or two old are most likely to respond to fibrinolytic therapy.

The most frequently used fibrinolytic agents are streptokinase and urokinase. Streptokinase is a nonenzymatic protein that is derived from beta-hemolytic streptococci (and therefore is antigenic to human beings). It combines with plasminogen to form a streptokinase-plasminogen complex; this converts plasminogen to plasmin, which in turn causes clot lysis. Streptokinase is generally administered at a relatively low rate (5000–10,000 U/hour) via an indwelling catheter embedded in the thrombus. The main disadvantages of strep-tokinase therapy are its antigenicity, the possibility that the patient's own antibodies to streptokinase may neutralize its effect, and its indirect activation of plasminogen.

Urokinase is a direct plasminogen activator that converts plasminogen to plasmin. Because it is derived from human fetal renal-cell cultures, it is not antigenic to human beings. Urokinase has been administered in both low- and high-dose protocols. In one recent study, a urokinase infusion of 4000 IU/min via a catheter embedded in the thrombus resulted in complete clot lysis in 83 percent of patients, with significant bleeding complications occurring in only 4 percent.

Patients undergoing fibrinolytic therapy should be monitored with serial determinations of fibrinogen level, fibrin degradation products, and of thrombin, prothrombin, and partial thromboplastin times. Ideally, the fibrinogen level should be kept above 100 mg/dL. Heparin is often administered concurrently in an effort to keep the partial thromboplastin time above 100 seconds. Infusion times range from 12 hours to several days. During this period, the patient should be closely monitored, preferably in an intensive care unit.

Further assessment of current fibrinolytic agents, as well as of newer agents such as tissue plasminogen activator, is essential for determining the proper role of fibrinolytic therapy in the treatment of arterial thrombosis.

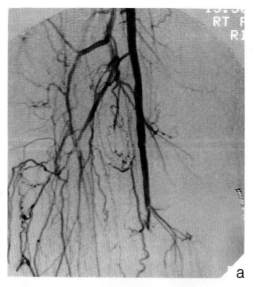
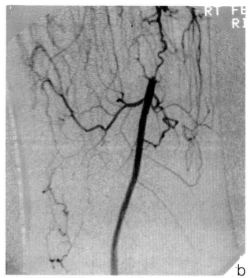

a

b

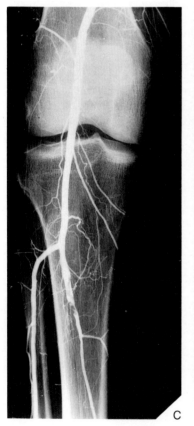
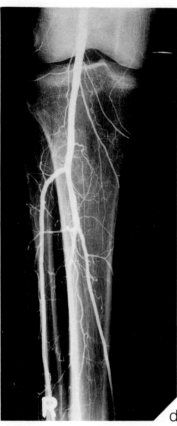

Fig. 12.8 Thrombolytic therapy.
*Three hours earlier, this patient experienced the sudden onset of pain and coldness in the right lower extremity. **a, b** A femoral arteriogram shows occlusion of a 5-cm segment of the superficial femoral artery as a result of a thromboembolus. Urokinase was infused through a catheter embedded in the embolus at a rate of 4000 IU/min. **c** A repeat arteriogram obtained after one hour of urokinase infusion no longer shows clot in the superficial femoral artery; however, thrombus fragments have migrated distally and lodged in the tibial-peroneal trunk. The catheter was then advanced into the tibial-peroneal trunk. **d** A repeat arteriogram following infusion of urokinase directly into the thrombus shows complete lysis of the thrombus.*

c

d

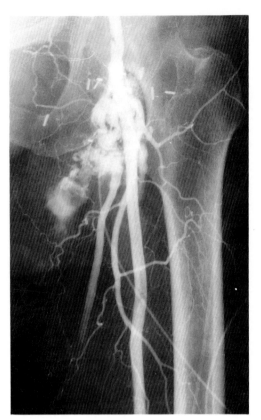

Fig. 12.9 Bleeding after transarterial thrombolysis. *A femoral arteriogram obtained after successful lysis of a clot in an occluded femoral-popliteal dacron graft shows extravasation of contrast material at the site of the proximal anastomosis. Bleeding is an occasional complication of transarterial thrombolysis.*

BIBLIOGRAPHY

Diagnostic Angiography

Abrams HL (ed.): *Angiography*, 3rd edn. Boston, Little, Brown & Co., 1983.

Athanasoulis CA, Pfister RC, Greene RE, Roberson GH (eds): *Interventional Radiology*. Philadelphia, WB Saunders, 1982.

Kadir S: *Diagnostic Angiography*. Philadelphia, WB Saunders, 1986. Neiman HL, Yao JST (eds): *Angiography of Vascular Disease*. New York, Churchill Livingstone, 1985.

Interventional Radiology

Droese M, Altmannsberger M, Kehl A, et al.: Ultrasound-guided percutaneous fine needle aspiration biopsy of abdominal and retroperitoneal masses. *Acta Cytol* 28(4):368–384, 1984.

Gunther RW, Schild H, Thelen M: Review article. Percutaneous transhepatic biliary drainage: experience with 311 procedures. *Cardiovasc Intervent Radiol* 11:65–71, 1988.

Keller FS, Rosch J, Dotter CT: Transhepatic obliteration of gastroesophageal varices with absolute ethanol. *Radiology* 146:615–619, 1983.

Lammer J, Neumayer K: Biliary drainage endoprostheses: experience with 201 placements. *Radiology* 159:625–629, 1986.

Lang EK, Price ET: Redefinition of indications for percutaneous nephrostomy. *Radiology* 147:419–426, 1983.

Mueller PR, Ferrucci JT, Teplick SK, et al.: Biliary stent endoprosthesis: analysis of complication in 113 patients. *Radiology* 156:637–639, 1985.

Mueller PR, von Sonnenberg E, Ferrucci JT: Percutaneous drainage of 250 abdominal abscesses and fluid collections. *Radiology* 151:343–347, 1984.

Mueller PR, von Sonnenberg E, Ferrucci JT, et al.: Biliary stricture dilatation: multicenter review of clinical management in 73 patients. *Radiology* 160:17–22, 1986.

Rahn NH, Tishler JM, Han SY, Russinovich N: Diagnostic and interventional angiography in acute gastrointestinal hemorrhage. *Radiology* 143:361–366, 1982.

Sigwart U, Puel J, Mirkovitch V, et al.: Intravascular stents to prevent occlusion and restenosis after transluminal angioplasty. N *N Engl J Med* 316(12):701–706, 1987.

Sos TA: Transhepatic portal venous embolization of varices: pros and cons. *Radiology* 148:569–570, 1983.

Steckman ML, Dooley MC, Jaques PF, Powell DW: Major gastrointestinal hemorrhage from peripancreatic blood vessels in pancreatitis. *Dig Dis Sci* 29(6), 1984.

Tegtmeyer C, Sos T: Techniques of renal angioplasty. *Radiology* 161:577–586, 1986.

Wold GL, LeVeen RF, Ring EJ: Potential mechanisms of angioplasty. *Cardiovasc Intervent Radiol* 7:11–17, 1984.

Zollikofer CL, Chain J, Salomonowitz E, et al.: Percutaneous transluminal angioplasty of the aorta. *Radiology* 151:355–363, 1984.

INDEX

Note: The numbers in **boldface** refer to Figure numbers.